Praise for
FIGHTING BACK

"A gift of inestimable value for parents and others concerned about the scourge of childhood sexual abuse. If only this book had been available when my children were young, I might have recognized the causes of my daughter's suffering—and been able to stop the abuse. It reveals the warning signs of a child or teen being lured or abused, how to talk to children about their safety in a nonjudgmental way, and how to get help. Kayla courageously shares how a survivor thinks about her experience and can heal from it."   —*Muriel T., Toronto, Canada*

"A much-needed look into a very complex topic that desperately needs to be addressed. As someone who personally experienced abuse, I know the isolation and shame it can bring. Reading Kayla's personal account, I had the feeling of being understood. My symptoms were a normal response to an abnormal situation. Although recovery is a long process, Kayla shows us that it is indeed possible. This book has the power to restore hope and save lives."   —*Cassandra P., Plymouth, Massachusetts*

"One of those rare books that will both capture your heart and feed your mind. The story of Kayla's personal struggle is painful and emotionally powerful. The timing of this book is perfect—our society needs to see these issues with the clarity and courage of Kayla Harrison and address them with the wisdom of Drs. Aguirre and Kaplan."
                    —*Bruce D. Perry, MD, PhD, Senior Fellow, The ChildTrauma Academy*

FIGHTING BACK

FIGHTING BACK

What an Olympic Champion's Story
Can Teach Us about Recognizing
and Preventing Child Sexual Abuse—
and Helping Kids Recover

KAYLA HARRISON,
Cynthia S. Kaplan, PhD,
and Blaise Aguirre, MD

THE GUILFORD PRESS
New York   London

Copyright © 2018 The Guilford Press
A Division of Guilford Publications, Inc.
370 Seventh Avenue, Suite 1200, New York, NY 10001
www.guilford.com

Printed in the United States of America

This book is printed on acid-free paper.

Last digit is print number: 9   8   7   6   5   4   3   2   1

The information in this volume is not intended as a substitute for consultation with healthcare professionals. Each individual's health concerns should be evaluated by a qualified professional.

Library of Congress Cataloging-in-Publication Data

Names: Harrison, Kayla, author. | Kaplan, Cynthia S. (Cynthia Sue) author. |
  Aguirre, Blaise A., author.
Title: Fighting back : what an Olympic champion's story can teach us about
  recognizing and preventing child sexual abuse— and helping kids recover /
  Kayla Harrison, Cynthia S. Kaplan, Blaise Aguirre.
Description: New York : The Guilford Press, 2018. | Includes bibliographical
  references and index.
Identifiers: LCCN 2017050490| ISBN 9781462532971 (paperback) |
  ISBN 9781462535699 (hardcover)
Subjects: LCSH: Child sexual abuse. | Abused children—Services for. | BISAC:
  FAMILY & RELATIONSHIPS / Abuse / Child Abuse. | BIOGRAPHY &
  AUTOBIOGRAPHY / Personal Memoirs. | PSYCHOLOGY / Psychotherapy /
  Child & Adolescent. | MEDICAL / Psychiatry / Child & Adolescent. |
  EDUCATION / Counseling / Crisis Management.
Classification: LCC HV6570 .H365 2018 | DDC 362.76—dc23
LC record available at *https://lccn.loc.gov/2017050490*

History, despite its wrenching pain, cannot be unlived,
But if faced with courage, need not be lived again.

—Maya Angelou

Contents

Authors' Note

To protect privacy, in many cases names of people in Kayla's story have been changed.

We alternate use of masculine and feminine pronouns, rather than using "he or she," for clarity and brevity.

Acknowledgments

Words cannot express our gratitude to The Guilford Press for believing in this project when it was little more than a good idea and several draft chapters. Specifically, our thanks go to Kitty Moore, our senior editor at Guilford, who took the time to patiently talk through all aspects of this undertaking and develop a vision for how best to convey Kayla's story and message. And then there is Chris Benton, our developmental editor, without whose professional advice, assistance, editing magic, and focus this book might well have stalled short of completion and certainly would not have been as well written and true to our mission. It is hard to capture the synergy that both Kitty and Chris contributed to this project, never veering from their commitment to our collective objective of reaching as large an audience as possible. Our goal is to raise awareness of child sexual abuse and the devastating toll it takes on its victims and to add our voices to those of others working toward the goal of preventing even one additional child from being hurt in this manner. Kitty and Chris were our champions and cheerleaders, and treated both the authors and the topic with the utmost respect and dignity. Thanks always.

And to the Pedros, who epitomize everything that coaches should be. They are true heroes, models of how power and influence can be used for good and the ways in which all adults can, and should, make a positive difference in the lives of the children they care for.

Of course we could not have done this without our families—our spouses and partners, who allowed us the time and space to work relentlessly when needed; Kayla's mom, who made brave contributions to the manuscript; and our collective children, who inspire us to make sure that society continues to make the protection of children the most sacred priority. And finally, we thank McLean Hospital, a relentless leader in the research and treatment of trauma, which provided us with the knowledge and experience necessary to help make this book a reality.

Prologue

November 2011

I can't sleep. I have been in Japan for 2 weeks, and every day I mentally mark another X on the calendar. It's November 2011, and I am 7 months away from competing in the Summer Olympics in London—a lifelong dream. For the most part, I can't sleep because I am anxious and can't wait to go home, but also because I am waiting for the bomb to drop, knowing that my secrets are about to be revealed to the world. Somewhere in the U.S., newspapers are being printed. Words are being typed. Not just any words. My words, my story, and I am scared to death.

I hadn't planned on talking about it. I never talked about it, not even with my closest friends. But something was in the air, something different. It took me a while to realize that what was different was me.

A month prior:

This reporter came into the dojo like all the others. She was very nice and reminded me of a mom; her name was Vicky. She greeted me and my coach, Jimmy, and then she and Jimmy went into his office to talk. I tried again to grasp the fact that USA Today had really sent her all the way from Colorado to talk to me. I was still so uncomfortable with the media attention I was receiving as the Olympics drew closer.

Jimmy and the reporter talked for quite a while, and then it was my turn. As we sat down and started talking, something happened; I immediately trusted Vicky in a way that was different from other interviewers. She was from USA Today after all—a national newspaper. We started with the typical judo questions—how old was I when I started, what drew me to judo, what did it feel like to be the fourth American to become a world champion. Blah blah blah. Then she stunned me with something that I wasn't expecting: "Jimmy alluded to the fact that you overcame a lot to get where you are. Would you like to share that with me?"

I paused and let it sink in. She wanted to go "there." I rarely went there, and I had certainly never gone there with someone from the media. I felt tears well up before I could calm myself down. My mind was racing. What should I say? "No comment"? That felt like such a stupid thing to say, and part of me did want to talk about it. The daily news was filled with stories of Penn State, Jerry Sandusky, and outrage for Joe Paterno. No reporters, however, were really placing their focus on the innocent children who had been victimized. I thought maybe no one cares about those kids—why is that? And then it hit me at that moment that maybe no one knows what it's like to be the victim and that maybe I could tell them . . . And so I did.

"Well . . . what Jimmy is talking about . . . I . . . I . . . I was sexually abused by my first coach. That's why I moved here." I stammered and cried through those words for the first time in a long time.

The rest of the interview was then all about that—about my climb up from the bottom. About my own personal hell and the people who had saved me, the people who changed my life forever. I told my story, and I cried, and she listened. She cried a little too. I talked and talked and talked; and when it was over we stepped out of the office and it was like a breath of fresh air. I closed that office door and felt like I had left behind at least a portion of the doubt, guilt, and hate that had haunted me for so very long. I felt so much lighter.

We hugged good-bye, and Vicky told me how proud she was of me. She said that the article would be published in November, and she would let me know the exact date. She wished me well in London and said she'd be watching.

I worked out that night and didn't think about a thing. I was just another judoka on the mat, striving toward that elusive Olympic gold. No one here had it, and I wanted it. That was my sole purpose; that was my goal. And it felt great.

I started talking publicly about my past so that I could help others. Help others find healing; help other victims know that they were not alone; and help those who hadn't experienced abuse begin to understand it. That first interview was one of the hardest and most rewarding things I have ever done. It was the day I started talking—and I haven't stopped since.

This book is a continuation of that effort. It is my hope and prayer that this book will help someone. It is my hope and prayer that this book will help many. Whether you have experienced a childhood trauma firsthand or not, it is my hope and prayer that you will read this book and see the issue of child sexual abuse with new eyes. It is my hope and prayer that you will tell someone what you have learned, that you will share this book with others, and that you will be educated and informed.

I still don't really know why I spilled my guts in that interview. Since then, however, I have witnessed again and again how the shame and guilt that victims feel works to perpetuate the problem. Abusers prey on that silence, and I've decided I will never again be part of that silence. I've decided that together, if more of us can break that silence sooner and others can recognize the warning signs of childhood abuse, this horror may just go away.

My name is Kayla Harrison. I am 27 years old. I am a world champion. I am America's first Olympic champion in judo. I am a friend. Sister. Daughter. Granddaughter. Student. Blonde. Jokester. Reader. Fighter. Mountain climber. Movie buff. Trivia maniac. Baseball fan. Shopaholic. I am all of these things and more. But this is not all I have been. I was a victim for a very long time, and now I am a Survivor.

Introduction

The sexual abuse of children impacts the most vulnerable members of society. It is widespread, affecting 1 in 7 girls by the age of 18 and 1 in 25 boys. Childhood sexual abuse (CSA) is not a new phenomenon; scientific reports date back to the mid-1800s. Nor is it limited to westernized cultures, as once believed. Yet the study of this enormously damaging public health problem is still in its infancy, public education about it is inadequate, and our children remain at grave risk.

Attention first became drawn to the problem of CSA in the 1960s and 1970s as the feminist political movement combined with the expansion of child welfare systems, allowing for the observation that sexual violence directed toward children was a large-scale problem that had been both underrecognized and undertreated. Then, during the latter half of the 20th century, the scope and nature of the problem was further highlighted by publicized incidents of child molestation, beginning with the "priest abuse" scandal that unfolded in the 1980s and extending to many high-profile cases of children sexually victimized by adult celebrities, athletes, coaches, and family members. The coverage of these incidents drew attention to the reality that our children are not at most risk from a stranger who hurts them on a single occasion as we once thought. Rather, the risk more than 75% (and many suggest as high as 90%) of the time is from an adult who knows the child and is often known to the child's family as well—someone who uses his power, access, and trust to begin to engage in sexual abuse.

We now have to grapple with the reality that the customary warnings about "stranger danger" are woefully inadequate to protect our children. What those of us who work with children hear time and time again from victims of child sexual abuse is that the person who sexually victimized them as a child was someone they, and often their family, trusted. We also hear that the abuse happened a little at a time and in secrecy and that, looking back, their biggest regret is not being fully forewarned about the realities of childhood sexual abuse—and that no one else in their life had noticed or asked at the time.

It is the stories of all of these victims who suffered in silence that led us to join together to write this book, a book we hope will serve as a cautionary tale for children and adults alike. As mental health professionals who have worked with child and adolescent victims of CSA for more than two decades, we (Dr. Kaplan and Dr. Aguirre) are acutely aware of the toll that childhood sexual maltreatment takes on a youth's well-being both in the short and longer term. Victims suffer from more depression, substance use, school failure, and other problems than their nonabused peers, and are significantly more likely to be revictimized as adults. More needs to be done to educate the public to recognize the signs that someone might be hurting a child and give both caregivers and youth knowledge and skills so they can identify and end sexual abuse as early as possible when it does occur.

We came together in writing this book to provide as much education as we can.

BLAISE AGUIRRE

I am a child and adolescent psychiatrist specializing in a condition known as borderline personality disorder (BPD). BPD is characterized by emotional extremes and relationship difficulties. Our research shows that nearly one-third of the patients we treat with BPD also have posttraumatic stress disorder (PTSD), and many of those are victims of childhood sexual abuse. We found that without treating the PTSD, particularly that caused by CSA, many patients, and their families, continued to suffer. Additionally, our patients often turned to self-harm in response to traumatic memories and experiences when they had no other coping skills.

Every child we treat has a parent or other adult caregiver, and part of the work we do is intended to develop the parents' capacity to see the world through their child's eyes and by so doing make better sense of their child's behavior. It is essential to teach parents about trauma, its impact and its treatment, and particularly the latest knowledge about scientifically sound and compassionate therapies, and so a large part of the work we do is educational.

Then given how often parents have either felt culpable or been blamed for their child's adversities, moving forward means ending the search for blame and fault, aiming instead to create the best lives possible for the young people we treat given the circumstances of their lives. In doing so, we empower ourselves to be better parents, caregivers, and human beings.

The privilege of working with my two coauthors has been its own reward. For the many years that I have known Cynthia Kaplan, she has been dedicated to the cause of CSA and PTSD. And I knew Kayla as a fierce competitor on the judo mat before I knew many of the details of her story. Today I know her as an even fiercer advocate for increasing awareness and reducing the stigma of CSA.

CYNTHIA KAPLAN

I am a child and adolescent psychologist who has spent my entire career working with individuals and families who have experienced trauma. Specifically my work has focused on childhood abuse and neglect and includes 25-plus years of helping CSA victims. This experience has taught me about the pain and emotional distress endured by children who are hurt by the very adults entrusted to care for them and the challenges these youth face when it comes to breaking their silence. So many times I have sat with children and teens who felt they could not speak up because they would be hurt or possibly not believed and that doing so might only "make matters worse." For every child I have treated there are often also distraught parents or caregivers who sit with me and bemoan their own lack of awareness and preparedness and express deep regret at not having recognized and stopped their loved one's abuse sooner.

Over the course of my career it has become increasingly clear that the solution to the problem of childhood abuse cannot come from treatment personnel alone, most of whom do not meet these victims until they are well into adolescence and adulthood and already bear the scars of their childhood trauma. Instead, those of us in this field must work together with victim advocates who have the best chance of persuading schools, communities, and legislatures about what needs to be done to stop this scourge. Kayla Harrison is just such an advocate, someone who refused to be silenced by her fear and shame and who found a way to reach out to me and Dr. Aguirre to ask if we would help tell her story in the hope that her first-person narrative would increase public awareness and prevention efforts and alert youth and adults alike to how CSA unfolds, goes unnoticed, and can be interrupted. Working with Kayla and Dr. Aguirre on this book has truly been a privilege and our collective and loving contribution to children, youth, and caregivers everywhere.

WHAT YOU CAN EXPECT FROM THIS BOOK

You may be a parent who has concerns about your own child. You could be a teacher, a school psychologist, a childcare worker, a babysitter, or a social worker. Perhaps you work in child protective services or the criminal justice system. In this book we are speaking to you, the individuals who are in close and regular contact with children and want to keep them safe. Our discussion includes children between the ages of 5 and 18, because these are the children we generally see in our practices and who are able to both recall and put words to their childhood experiences of sexual abuse. That is not to say that younger children are not traumatized, as there are certainly many corroborated reports of infants and preschool-age children being subjected to abuse that they may not themselves recall or be able to dialogue about; many of these cases come to the attention of child protective services and legal services and are beyond the scope of this book. While most of the information and advice we give applies broadly to all forms of CSA, including incest (and we have noted some additional considerations about incest), this is a complicated separate topic that we cannot do justice to in this book, and we offer additional sources of information and help in the Resources appendix.

This book would not be possible without Kayla Harrison's brave revelations of the sexual abuse she suffered at the hands of her coach; it is these firsthand accounts that give all of us a chance to see explicitly how CSA can begin, persist, and be brought to an end. In the chapters that follow, we trace the course of Kayla's victimization and survival, weaving her story with our professional experience with hundreds of children, teens, and families to reveal what can be done to prevent and interrupt this damaging cycle. Essentially the chapter order matches the chronology of child sexual abuse, from the point when a child is targeted by a perpetrator to the child's ultimate recovery from being victimized in this devastating way.

- The first three chapters set the stage, describing how abusers groom a potential victim, why and how children stay silent—often for a very long time—and what creates the critical tipping point where disclosure finally becomes possible.

- The next three chapters explain what you can expect after a child's sexual abuse is revealed and how to handle this difficult period to offer the utmost protection to a child who has already been severely harmed: what to anticipate from the legal system and how to prepare and support the child, how to help the child manage the longer-term emotional effects, and how to use state-of-the-art professional help to ease and hasten the recovery process.

- Finally, in the last two chapters we show what recovery can look like and how to get there. In these pages you'll hear about what victims, doctors, therapists, and researchers have found most helpful to children and teens on their journey to the life they always deserved to have. You'll also learn about education and advocacy initiatives and institutions that offer help throughout the country—and how you, as Kayla has, can support and promote these programs, as well as using these resources to help any victimized children in your own life.

It's important to understand before you start reading, however, that the course of child sexual abuse is not entirely linear. Events and developments are often intertwined, and although we have organized these chapters to make information easy to understand and retain—and refer back to as needed—topics covered in one chapter may very well take shape and affect the child and family at the same time as those discussed in the next chapter. We strongly encourage reading the entire book to get a complete understanding of this problem and its solutions.

We hope you will emerge from reading this book with a better understanding of how perpetrators gain access to and violate children in secrecy, along with a sharper ability to recognize what may be happening to children you care about. We hope you will also learn how to respond effectively to help these victims through the difficult aftermath of disclosing their abuse and when and how to access professional mental health help as needed. Finally, we offer hope through understanding the recovery process—how children can make the transition from victim to survivor, as Kayla has, and find a path to a meaningful life.

1

How Child Sexual Abuse Begins

I started judo when I was 6 years old. My mother took judo in college, and so when I was little she wanted me to learn self-defense. I think she also wanted to get me out of the house a little bit because I was kind of a wild child. From the very beginning I loved it. I loved everything about it. Bowing at the beginning of every class to show respect. Learning how to throw people through the air, and even learning how to fall and fly through the air properly so that I didn't get hurt were cool tricks to show my friends at recess. And most of all, judo made me feel special. It was the thing I did, I realize now looking back, that made me different from everyone else. And I loved that.

When I first started judo, though, I wasn't very good. In fact, I didn't win a match for the first year of competition. In judo, the object is to score ippon, which is like a knockout in boxing. There are four ways to score ippon:

- By pinning your opponent for 20 seconds
- By choking your opponent until she concedes by tapping the floor (for 13 years and older)
- By arm barring your opponent until she taps out (for 15 years and older)
- By throwing your opponent flat on her back

7

Well, in my first year of competition I kept finding myself flat on my back with the referee calling "ippon" for the other girls. First I would only last 15 seconds in a match, and then I made it a whole minute. Finally, I lasted a whole match and didn't lose by ippon, just by points. And then the day finally came that I'll never forget.

I was about 8 years old and at a local tournament in Indiana (I grew up in southern Ohio). The tournament was by no means a big one. A small high school gymnasium was filled with judo mats and parents, mostly moms, with their kids. Maybe 300 people in total. I probably only had three girls in my division, but I beat those three girls and I won. I won the whole thing. And then it was my turn to stand on top of the podium, and I received a trophy that was as big as me.

And I knew—I knew right then. I didn't want to be a singer or a doctor. I didn't want to be an actress; I wanted to throw people. And I wanted to be the best in the world at it. But being the best in the world at anything isn't easy. You need the right team.

So shortly after I won and started competing more whole-heartedly, I told my mom I wanted to train in earnest, by which I meant at that time that I wanted to go to judo more to see my friends. My mom would also tell me if I enjoyed winning and wanted more trophies I would have to train for them, which I was all too eager to do! There was a club about 45 minutes from us that was a much more competitive club, and we agreed that I would start going there and see how things went.

Walking into the Renshuden Judo Academy for the first time was overwhelming. I was so scared! My little judo class in Hamilton was in a school, and there were only a couple kids in the class, and they were mostly kids my age with not a lot of experience. At Renshuden I saw all ages and ranks on the mat: black belts, purple belts, teenagers, and blue belts. I think at the time I was a green belt and not a very experienced one at that. I could tell right away, however, that I was definitely going to like it there.

The head sensei, or teacher, was a little Irish man with twinkling eyes and a smile on his face. I liked him right away. And although the kids seemed intimidating, they also were eager to help me learn. Right away they started showing me stuff and helping me with my uchikomi, or the practice of my throws. By the end of the very first class when it was time to bow out and go home

I was hooked. I couldn't wait to go back and learn with all of my new friends.

Not long after I started at Renshuden, Daniel, the head sensei's son, came home from training in Scotland and I immediately knew that I wanted him to like me and that he could help me be the best in the world at judo . . . and so my relationship with Daniel began.

What Kayla, at the age of 8, could not have known was that Daniel could not be trusted. Kayla, like most children this age, still looked at coaches, teachers, and adults in general as people who could be counted on—counted on to behave in a predictable and honorable fashion. It is this trust that child predators prey on as they first earn, and then abuse, the faith placed in them by a child. And it is their very importance and prestige that makes it possible to earn not only the confidence of the child but also often the confidence of the child's family. Once this trust is established, it is only a small step for individuals with dishonorable intentions to first isolate and then begin to inappropriately touch a child in their care. This is how child sexual abuse (CSA) happens, and this process must be more fully understood if we are to more effectively protect youth everywhere.

WHAT EXACTLY IS CHILD SEXUAL ABUSE?

The definition of child sexual abuse may seem obvious, but its classification as a condition of interest to mental health professionals and a punishable crime is shockingly recent. It was not until the late 1970s that a majority of states in the United States had mandatory reporting laws that required adults with knowledge of CSA to tell child welfare and legal authorities.

For the purposes of this book we are using the American Psychiatric Association's 2013 definition, which is essentially that CSA is any sexual behavior engaged in by any adult that involves a person under the age of consent and is designed to be sexually gratifying to that adult. The legal definition is essentially the same, although the letter of the law varies from state to state (and is discussed further in

To find out how your state defines child sexual abuse in the applicable civil and criminal statutes, go to *www.childwelfare.gov/ topics/systemwide/laws- policies/state.*

Chapter 4). For the purposes of this book we are defining a "child" as someone under 18 years of age.

Child sexual abuse can take many forms—including both touching and nontouching behaviors (from the Hero Project):

Touching behaviors include but are not limited to:

- Fondling or touching a child's genitals for sexual pleasure or other unnecessary reasons.

- Making or inducing a child to touch someone else's genitals.

- Penetration of the vulva or vagina, the mouth, or the anus of a child by the perpetrator for sexual pleasure or other unnecessary reason.

Nontouching sexual behaviors include but are not limited to:

- Exposing a child to, or using a child for the purpose of prostitution.

- Performing sexual acts in a child's presence.

- Photographing a child in sexual poses and/or exposing the child to pornography.

- Watching a child undress or use the bathroom, often without the child's knowledge.

- Using computers and the internet to make sexual overtures or expose a child to sexual behavior.

- Indecent exposure.

Child sexual abuse typically begins gradually, and perpetrators of child sexual abuse can spend months "grooming" a victim with nonsexual hugging and touching—behavior that at first seems perfectly normal and acceptable. When the behavior becomes increasingly sexual, the child is most often confused, frightened, and feels powerless to make it stop. As you will see through the excerpts written from Kayla Harrison's personal experiences with sexual abuse, the child victim may want to be special in some way to the adult—a specialness that the perpetrator then takes advantage of as he incrementally trades his attention and affection for escalating sexual favors.

WHAT WE KNOW ABOUT SEXUAL ABUSERS OF CHILDREN

Not that long ago, the prevailing assumption was that the people who abused or hurt children would be obvious in some way, conjuring up for many a creepy man lurking at the edge of a school playground or prowling the bushes and parks. This, however, has not turned out to be accurate since, according to almost all studies and evidence we now have, sexual abusers are most often the people that our children know, often someone parents feel close to and someone the child cares about and trusts.

Because sexual abuse of a child is so abhorrent, the idea of the abuser as an unknown—and unknowable—pervert can seem easier to accept than the truth: Many abusers are family members or family friends, teachers and day care providers, neighbors, babysitters, religious leaders or coaches and, thus, are the very people who are in close, unsupervised contact with children on a daily basis. In fact, among victims of sexual abuse that draw the attention of law enforcement, studies reliably indicate that more than a quarter are victimized by a family member, while 60% are abused by someone else from their social network. Research by Howard Snyder and Melissa Sickmund of the National Center for Juvenile Justice showed that only 14% are victimized by someone they did not already know (see the box on page 12 for more data on CSA perpetrators).

> Reports from the National Institutes of Justice (2003) and other governmental agencies indicate that more than three out of four of the adolescents in the United States who have been sexually assaulted were victimized by someone they knew well.

Unfortunately these findings confirm that personal appearance, public behavior, or occupation will not serve as clues to who among us is a potential abuser. When identifying a child abuse risk, it's not who a person is—his age, position, gender, or ascribed status in a community—that matters; it's how that adult chooses to interact with the children under his or her care or supervision. What we do know is that sexual abuse happens universally and that perpetrators most often gain access to a child in a manner that does not initially arouse suspicion in adults or fear in the child. This means that people who sexually abuse children typically don't appear outwardly dangerous. The fact that they can be the very people we feel most trusting of and

---

WHO SEXUALLY ABUSES CHILDREN AND TEENS?

According to Statistics on Perpetrators of CSA (2017):

- Contrary to popular beliefs, perpetrators of CSA are not all male; it's estimated that women are the abusers in about 14% of cases reported among boys and 6% of cases reported among girls.
- About a third of perpetrators are other children or teens.
- About 60% of abusers are in the victim's social circle.
- Somewhere between a third and a half of sexually abused girls are victimized by a family member; the rate is much lower (10–20%) for abused boys.
- Of those molesting a child under age 6, 50% are family members.

---

familiar with is often instrumental in their securing access to their victims.

For a parent or anyone else charged with the care of children, these facts can be terrifying. How can you protect your son or daughter or student if the perpetrator of sexual abuse is likely to be someone you are inclined to trust? The answer is that the greatest degree of protection comes from knowing the behaviors that may be a red flag that an individual is beginning to interact or treat a child in inappropriate ways that may signal the beginning of what we refer to as "grooming," often the introductory phase of sexual abuse.

As was true for Kayla's mother and stepfather, many parents of abused children never thought that an adult who was presumably helping their child might simultaneously be taking advantage of his status and access to that child. Kayla's mother described to her how their family was seduced by the help Daniel offered: "He was always saying stuff about your potential and about the Olympics. He wanted you to make the Olympic trials when you were 13. Your dad and I stayed in a timeshare, and you stayed with the team in a hotel. Because of the Olympic dream, there was a lot of behavior that I did not question. Even to the point when we thought about moving you to the national training center with Jimmy but Daniel said no, he could coach you, and we believed him. You also had a fit and did not want to leave. You were very insistent that you were getting good training where you were and you didn't want to leave. And Daniel was as well. He always said that your potential was amazing. And I always thought that too. I always went to the ends of the earth to make sure you reached your potential."

Disbelief about the possibility of abuse is particularly strong when the perpetrator is a family member, and finding out about incest is perhaps the hardest type of sexual abuse for other family members to accept. Kayla's mother had believed that Daniel's behavior, even when harsh, represented his efforts to help Kayla rather than hurt her and had accepted him in essence as a member of the family with all of the trust and access that this designation carries. In an interview after Daniel's abuse of her daughter was revealed, Kayla's mom talked about her general lack of awareness and her assumption that abuse is not something perpetrated by family friends or other trusted adults:

> "Daniel became a trusted family friend. He babysat all three of our children . . . they all would spend the night at his house. He went on vacations with us because our vacations were around judo. He was a member of the family.
>
> "I was devastated and horrified when I heard from Kayla that Daniel had sexually abused her. I can't imagine that I didn't know. Still, it's just something I never thought could really happen. There are days that I still think, 'How in the world could I not have known?'"

WHAT WE KNOW ABOUT GROOMING BEHAVIOR

Sexual predators often *groom* their victims for abuse behavior. The grooming process begins with the abuser identifying a child who seems vulnerable. We now know that some abusers look for children who have low self-esteem or lack confidence, are lonely, or are in need of attention (see the box on page 14). But just as often the abuser is someone who has access to the targeted child and the power to provide or withhold things the child needs. This is what gives relatives, teachers, caregivers, and coaches so much potential for misusing their authority—gradually beginning to violate a child's boundaries without discovery or repercussion.

The first time I met Daniel he was on the mat running around and playing with all my new friends. The first thing I remember about him was how fun he was. At 6'1" and 230 pounds, he was an adult and a black belt but always wanted to play games with us and goof off. His bald head and big belly gave him away as a grown man, though.

More often than not Daniel's father would spend half the class yelling at Daniel to knock it off! It was always a fun atmosphere, but everyone there trained hard. And the more time I spent at Daniel's home, the more I wanted Daniel to notice me. He definitely had his favorites, and although he could be harsh to them and it scared me, I also noticed they were the best in the class, and I wanted that so badly.

Selecting Vulnerable Victims

Taken together, what we know from studying the characteristics of child victims and direct reports from perpetrators is that they actively look for children who are passive and may be lonely or troubled due to larger family circumstances, such as coming from single-parent or broken homes. They also look for services or tangible items they can offer a child or family to increase access and reliance.

RISK FACTORS FOR BEING TARGETED FOR SEXUAL ABUSE

From *Darkness to Light* (2017):

- Family structure: not having both biological parents in the home
- Gender: girls are five times more likely than boys to be sexually abused
- Age: greatest risk from ages 7 to 13 (median age is 9)
- Low socioeconomic status and being a member of a racial or ethnic minority group
- Low self-esteem or confidence; passive
- Loneliness or isolation
- A need for attention or specific types of help that the perpetrator can provide
- Eagerness to please

Expanding the Relationship

After selecting a child, based in part on the child's unsuspecting willingness to engage and in part on the child's falling into the vulnerability categories given in the box on page 14, the abuser commonly forms an expanded relationship with the child that is substantively different from a "normal" adult–child relationship, although, again, the perpetrator typically attempts to make the relationship appear "normal" when others are around. The perpetrator gradually begins to demand acts and behaviors from the child that become obligatory if the child wants this person's ongoing favor, approval, and protection. This process can be seen in Kayla's recollections from that early time as she began to work harder to gain Daniel's admiration:

Daniel terrified me. He was unlike anyone I'd ever met before. Not caring and understanding like my family and friends but harsh—insatiable. And satisfying him quickly became my sole purpose. Slowly at first, because honestly, for a while, I'm sure I wasn't even on his radar. And why should I have been? I was mediocre at best. The fear suppressed any bursts of ability that I had. And the raw talent all around me didn't help. Used to being the star in the context of the general pool of kids my age, I was unaccustomed to being looked over, to being just another someone.

But this new obstacle affected me in several different ways. Sometimes my confidence and self-esteem would dip so low I would become a mere mirage of the child I truly was. Other times my "normalness" would infuriate me to the point of explosion. I can recall nights of endless tears full of frustration and fear. I wasn't used to failing. And I wasn't used to people I wanted to admire me, treating me with indifference. This, ultimately, changed my path. My failure became my fuel.

Kayla believes that she was particularly vulnerable to Daniel's abuse because she was naturally inclined to try to please others, and in fact this is not unusual. Research by Helen Whittle and colleagues shows that abuse, intermixed with small acts of tenderness and generosity by the abuser, can bond some victims to their abuser. Children eager to please their abuser are particularly vulnerable:

I do feel looking back as if my mentality and natural disposition made me more of a "target" for sexual abuse. I always wanted to *please. Whether this meant staying after class and rebinding books for my sixth-grade teacher or pushing myself to limits of exhaustion for a coach, I have always had that "I will be the best" mentality. I have always felt "special" in that sense. I trusted the Pedros [Kayla's later coaches in Boston] as much as I trusted Daniel, but the results were <u>completely</u> different because they were not predators. I think it was a matter of having an athlete who is willing to sacrifice so much (often from an extremely young age because when you have that mentality it doesn't matter how young or old you are) and having it exploited by the right person when I was at an age that I didn't understand if it was right or wrong or okay. I was only sure that I loved judo, I loved Daniel, and so I must do this because that is what people in love and people who are successful do.*

Not all children have a special talent or need that the abuser is satisfying, as with Kayla. In many cases the expanded relationship involves the perpetrator simply using the difference in power between the child and a parent, clergy, or caregiver to initiate sexual contact. From what we know about the intentions and thinking of child perpetrators, they often target a child because of both attraction and accessibility.

Getting the Child Used to Touch

Once a child has been chosen, the abuser typically begins to gradually desensitize the child to touch, making it a standard aspect of their relationship and an integral part of the child's ensuring ongoing preferred status with the abuser. The first contact between predator and victim is often nonsexual touching—an "accidental" touch or an arm around a shoulder. There might be a lot of tickling and physical play. Once the child gets used to being touched, the abuser advances to touching in other ways. The boundaries between appropriate and inappropriate touching are purposely blurred. When necessary, the abuser reassures the child that the transactions are positive and special.

Examples of common grooming activities include:

- Pulling down a child's underwear without permission.
- Holding a child on the perpetrator's lap while having an erection.
- Kissing the child in a way that is sexual for the perpetrator.

- Forms of seemingly harmless touching, cuddling, wrestling, tickling, or playing that have sexual overtones or meaning for the perpetrator.

- Treating a child as an equal or peer or like a spouse by giving the child gifts or taking him or her places that are out of the ordinary, such as giving necklaces or taking the child to mature-rated movies.

Getting used to nonsexual touching and being treated in what first seems to be a "special" fashion weakens a child's natural inhibitions and defenses, and once the child does not resist such contact, the abuser tends to escalate to more sexual touching. In Kayla's case, this desensitization began with Daniel's assuming a more central role in her training. In judo, this naturally involves a great deal of necessary physical contact between student and coach. As she describes this early phase of her relationship with the man who would go on to abuse her, Kayla clearly is unsuspecting of any underlying or inappropriate motives on Daniel's part:

Over time, Daniel started to help me more and more. He even gave me a nickname, which at the time I didn't know was a little mean. "Chunky Monkey" became my name. I was so proud when he called me that. I was special enough to deserve a nickname. I was somebody!

Jon Conte, Steven Wolf, and Tim Smith, in their classic article "What Sexual Offenders Tell Us About Prevention Strategies," presented results from a series of interviews with 20 child sexual offenders who shared what they did to engage the child in sexual contact as they entered into the grooming process. These interviews shed important light on how insidious and intentional these individuals' efforts are in targeting an individual child.

"Talking, spending time with them, being around them at bedtime, being around them in my underwear, sitting down on the bed with them. Constantly evaluating the child's reaction . . . A lot of touching, hugging, kissing, snuggling."

"Playing, talking, giving special attention, trying to get the child to initiate contact with me . . . Get the child to feel safe to talk with me . . . From here I would initiate different kinds of contact, such as touching the child's back, head . . . Testing the child to see how much she would take before she would pull away."

"Isolate them from other people. Once alone, I would make a game of it (red light, green light with touching up their leg until they said stop). Making it fun."

"It's Our Little Secret"

At some point during the grooming process a child predator will introduce an element of secrecy. This not only strengthens the child's trust in and reliance on the adult but also starts to isolate the child, distancing her parents and other surrounding adults. The predator may start by allowing the child to do something small that a parent might not approve of—eating candy, staying up late, engaging in risky or forbidden behaviors, and the like. Once the abuser has escalated to inappropriate, sexualized touching, he will commonly use manipulation and threats of various degrees to stop the child from telling if the child expresses displeasure or concern. Most typically the abuser will:

- Tell the child that the contact is "our little secret."
- Tell the child that telling someone else would get them both in trouble.
- Tell the child that no one will believe her even if she does tell.
- Threaten the child with the loss of the entire relationship if he tells.

In some cases there is even the threat of physical retaliation against both the child and the family. As Kayla now remembers, Daniel worked hard to make sure that she believed that her success and well-being depended entirely on his beneficence, threatening her with the loss of their relationship were she to question his control, advice, or conduct:

> To ensure I believed that success was only possible with him, Daniel would do little things. Cut me down in front of others, make me feel insecure and isolated. Make me feel like my judo was horrible and the only way I could get better was through him. It got to the point where I wanted and needed his approval over anyone's: my parents, my family, my friends . . . they all played second fiddle to being in his

good graces. At the same time he was very smart about giving praise and showing signs of affection. If I did good at a tournament, he would let me sit in his lap on the often-long drive home and rub my back. Or he would let me play in the pool with him and climb on him. He would criticize and push me but then make it so that only he could build me back up. It was a spot of honor to sit next to Daniel in the car or at a team dinner. It was a big deal if you worked hard enough to earn a "good job" from him. They were rare at best.

At the same time, he was very much one of us. He would have sleepovers at his house and let us drink with him. He would swim with us in the hotel pools when none of the other adults would and play silly juvenile games with the boys and me. He was both terrifying in the power he had over us and heartwarming in his role as equal.

The threat of falling out of Daniel's "good graces" and losing the relationship with him in turn pushed Kayla, like so many child victims, to work harder to please her abuser even at the cost of other close relationships. In fact, it's a central part of the grooming process for the victim's family and social circle first to accept the abuser's relationship as appropriate, only to find later that they have been gradually replaced by the abuser in terms of influence over the child. This happened with Kayla as she spent increasing amounts of time alone with Daniel:

Things changed slowly at first. I began to receive more attention; I realize now that it wasn't really me. His star pupils were fading. Every day it seemed as if another student was dropping out to start another sport or getting a boyfriend. This resulted in his more urgent need for me. I wasn't as dispensable as before. I realize now that my success was partially a symptom of his attention, not a cause.

Nevertheless, things continued to progress little by little. He began to push me just a little bit harder at practice. He was often brutal and savage. But unlike most of his pupils, who cowered away from this, I reveled in it. I had never experienced anything quite like him. He was rude and hurtful and never satisfied. Of course this fueled me.

My sole purpose was to appease and satiate those around me. From a young age I was always a pleaser. I feel as if it played right *into his hand. I cared so much about what others, especially adults, thought of me. I was always a teacher's pet and a role model student. I was well beloved by all my coaches, not just Daniel. He was the only one who took that and made it into something abusive.*

I withdrew myself from all outside life and focused solely on him and our goals as a team. Daniel could do no wrong in my eyes.

Our bond was already strengthened by the time my family began to worry, and instead of listening I rebelled. Strongly. He became my only ally. My only friend. And that's pretty much when it started in earnest.

By the time I was 11 years old I was Daniel's favorite. The relationship had been inappropriate for some time, and the more successful I became the more toxic the relationship became. By 12 I was Junior National Champion, I was beginning to fight in the senior divisions (the divisions that qualify for the Olympics), and I was winning more and more. I was also shutting down from the rest of my life. No hanging out with non-judo friends, no more nice clothes, which I had always loved shopping for with my Mimi (my mom's mother). No more spending quality time with my family. I was becoming a different person. Successful and confident in judo but a mess inside and emotionally. Very unstable. And Daniel created that havoc and that change in me in order to isolate and capitalize on my success as an athlete, my desire to win, and my willingness to do anything and be whoever I needed to be in order to do so.

Instilling Guilt

Often, the final step in the grooming process is to make the child feel like the abuse is her fault. Victims often believe that they did something to cause the abuse to start in the first place or that, by not fighting back physically or saying "no," they somehow let the abuse happen. This can be very confusing, leaving the child feeling guilty. Many abused children later describe feeling like a *co-conspirator* with the perpetrator. They may believe that their silence allowed the abuse to continue. Some, like many teens we've worked with, even become convinced that they acted "seductively" as a young child or failed to behave as expected in some other fashion, thus causing the sexual abuse to begin and continue. Kayla describes an increasing awareness, as the contact with Daniel became more sexualized, that she had to keep this aspect of their relationship a secret or risk losing everything that was important to her—judo, Daniel, and the very "specialness" that she had come to crave:

Some days, he would only play with me on the mat and teach me special moves. But eventually, as I look back, it is clear that things would get gradually more and more sexual.

On days when I would be sitting on the couch doing my homework he would come over and rub my back or sit next to me and rub my knee or tickle me.

Then on days when he was tired he would lie down with his sunglasses on and have me lie in his lap while he rubbed my back.

But no matter what, he would always have one eye open for someone coming to the dojo. He would always sit up or scoot away from me before anyone else ever came through the door, and that made me feel funny.

I knew (fairly quickly) that what was happening between us was our secret, and I knew I shouldn't tell anyone, especially if I wanted to remain special. That made me feel funny too.

Trapping the Child in Silence

By this point in the grooming process, it is in most cases impossible for the victim to take steps to end the relationship with the abuser, and it's up to other adults in the child's family and social circle to take notice of the increasing isolation, dependency, and anxiety that accompany the child's relationship with this specific adult. This can be particularly challenging if the abuser is at that point a beloved and trusted individual. The adult's behavior has likely changed so gradually that it goes unsuspected and undetected without further vigilance.

Signs That a Child May Be Trapped in an Abusive Relationship

Some of the signs that parents later tell us they noticed without recognizing their significance include:

- The child begins to focus almost solely on one activity and/or one adult.
- The child begins to show unexplained fear of or unwillingness to talk about a specific adult.

- The child begins to talk and worry about a specific adult in her life.
- The child stops showing interest in other activities and people she typically likes.
- The child becomes significantly less willing to talk about a specific activity or adult.
- The child decreases social activity, except with respect to a specific activity/adult.

Kayla's judo commitments obscured the fact that the increased opportunity for contact between her and Daniel had taken a more sinister turn:

By the time I was 9 or 10 I started traveling with the team to local tournaments. After being at Daniel's dad's gym for about 2 years, I was allowed to start spending more time with them and having team sleepovers.

At night, when the whole team would watch movies, I would snuggle up next to him. He would put a blanket over us, and then one day things went further and he guided my hand to touch him. I didn't really understand what it meant, but I knew he liked it, and I wanted to please him, so I did it.

What's the lesson for parents and other caregivers here? *The best way to recognize grooming behaviors is to pay very close attention to your child and the people in your child's life. Do not unquestioningly surrender responsibility for your children to other adults, no matter how reasonable it may seem initially, without asking questions and maintaining a level of watchful supervision.*

It's also important to realize, however, that a child sexual predator recognizes that conditioning or convincing the child not to tell another adult is not going to be enough to avoid discovery. The perpetrator must also go to lengths to persuade other adults of his trustworthiness with children. It's this entire process—the seduction of the child along with involvement with the parent/caregiver in a child's environment—that constitutes grooming and that typically occurs in up to 90% of instances in which the perpetrator is already an acquaintance of the child before the abuse begins.

> Grooming involves seduction of the family along with the child.

How You Can Increase the Likelihood of Noticing That Something Is Wrong

There are no easy answers or foolproof solutions, but there are some steps that parents, caregivers, educators, and professionals can take:

- Monitor the amount of time a child spends alone with any particular adult and notice any increase or change in this pattern.
- Talk with the child directly about any "special" relationships she develops with a trusted adult in her environment.
- Look for any shift in which the child isolates himself from friends and family, opting instead to spend time with a specific adult.
- Closely monitor situations in which adults assume significant control and power over a child's success, such as in sports, school, and religious domains.
- If you begin to worry about a specific relationship, increase the amount of involvement of other parents, adults, and peers to decrease the opportunity for isolation and secrecy.
- If you notice clear signs that a child may be engaged in an inappropriate relationship with an adult, don't be afraid to let both the child and adult know of your suspicions.

Grooming the Family

Many predators will even try to gain access to children by grooming the parents first. For example, an abuser may pretend to be interested in dating the mother, but is really interested in her daughter. Likewise, a trusted teacher or coach may offer to tutor or otherwise help a child for no fee, with the hidden agenda of gaining isolated yet sanctioned access to that child. Especially for children who become involved in elite athletics, music, or academics, their coach or mentor holds a great deal of power based on having expertise that a parent does not. This competitive control over the child is highlighted in Kayla's description of fallout, involving both her mother and Daniel, over dyeing her hair:

> We were on a trip to New Mexico the first time he did anything that made me really feel uncomfortable. We were at a Junior

National tournament, and the whole team was there. My mom was with me and I think my sister too.

I remember this trip was especially awful for me because Daniel was very angry with me. My friend Lisa had dyed her hair purple before the competition, and I wanted to do something crazy too. So I asked my mom, and she said I could. Well, Lisa dyed my hair red for me! It was going to be a big surprise, and I thought Daniel would love it.

But when we picked him up at the airport, he was furious with my mother, and I remember him yelling at my mom, saying nasty things about how it looked and telling her I could be disqualified from the tournament if the dye came out of my hair.

I was terrified and made my mom take me to the drugstore and, right then and there at the hotel the night before my big competition, I bleached all the color out of my hair so Daniel wouldn't be mad at me anymore.

I hated how it looked, but it was better than Daniel being mad at me. I would do just about anything to avoid that. That night I sheepishly walked into the room where everyone was watching a movie. I kept my eyes down, and no one said a word about my hair. I think we were all afraid Daniel would get angry again.

I went to sit down on the floor in front of the TV, and Daniel called for me. "Chunky Monkey, come sit by me," he said. All the air went out of my lungs I was so relieved. If I got to sit by him, that must mean he wasn't mad anymore and my bleaching of my hair had worked.

I jumped on the bed and climbed over to him. He put his arm around me and whispered to me, "Blondes always have more fun." I giggled and looked up at him. He was so silly, and I would dye my hair for the rest of my life if it meant he wasn't mad at me.

This scenario paints a stark picture of the way in which Daniel had gradually assumed authority and control over Kayla and, in a sense, over her family as well. These power shifts happen gradually, and it's easy for parents and other adults in the child's life to respond by acquiescing rather than challenging or questioning them. As suggested by the founders of the Hero Project—a multimedia campaign, initiated in 2010, challenging adults to be heroes for children they suspected were being abused by calling the Pennsylvania Coalition

Against Rape's hotline—and echoed by other organizations focused on expanding awareness of the grooming process:

> Parents should know their child's teachers, coaches, day care providers, youth group leaders, and other significant adults in their lives. Make unannounced visits. Ask questions. Stay involved. It is all very important to keep the lines of communication open with your child. Teach him/her to tell you about any physical contact initiated by an adult and to trust you with problems and emotions. Let him/her know that he/she can talk to you about problems and concerns without you reacting and getting angry.

A GRADUAL, INSIDIOUS, ESCALATING BETRAYAL

This review of the grooming process reveals how targeted and intentional these behaviors are in most cases. Not only does the perpetrator most often know the child victim, but much of the time the grooming process is gradual and well planned, designed to blind both the child and other concerned adults to the perpetrator's intentions.

Recognizing when a trusted adult is beginning to act inappropriately and gradually violate the boundaries of a relationship is quite difficult for almost all children and younger teens; they are reeled in a little at a time to trust that what is going on is "okay" even though they may suspect it is not. This trust in a significant and possibly important adult in their lives is often further bolstered by the parallel trust and access afforded the perpetrator, unknowingly, by the victim's family and friends. Because the relationship looks special and feels special and can often give the victim and parents tangible advantages—from free tutoring to time off, extra coaching, or money—the grooming process is seductive to the entire family system constellation.

Kayla's mother recalled to Kayla how Daniel seduced their family:

> "He was always thoughtful. He would show up at the hospital when you were sick to check on you. I thought it was because he cared, but now I know it was because he wanted to make sure you didn't say anything. I always thought he cared about your well-being. But now I know he never wanted you too far out of reach.
> "I feel like now if a coach or someone close to your child is overly interested or concerned, then perhaps you should look into

the relationship a little further. But there should be boundaries, and if you sense they are hovering you need to be aware that the relationship may be bordering on the line of inappropriate.

"He really integrated himself into our lives, and I think that people should be wary of coaches or professionals doing that."

It is the proverbial wolf in sheep's clothing that we have most to fear, and it is the grooming process that ensnares nearly all child victims and their families. This alarming progression is described by Kayla as she recalls the escalation of her relationship with Daniel:

After a while the lights went out and the movie got longer and longer, or so it seemed. About half way through he pulled the covers up over us both and started touching me under the blanket.

I always got scared when he did this because I didn't want any-one to see us.

A little bit later he started to pull my underwear to the side and try to put his finger in me. I was so shocked I remember I tried to stop his hand and started crying a little because I didn't like it and I was getting scared.

But he seemed to not be mad and he pushed harder when I tried to stop him. He leaned into me and said, "This is our secret, baby," . . . and I let him.

When the movie ended I went into the bathroom and cried. I felt so dirty and so gross I didn't even want to look at myself in the mirror. But I knew I loved Daniel, and I knew this is what people in love do so I closed my eyes and I said to myself to be a big girl and stop crying like a baby.

This is what you wanted. But it wasn't. And I had no idea it was only going to get worse.

Kayla's story is typical of that of many children who are sexu-ally abused: most know and trust the adults who later abuse them. Whether with a clergy member, coach, mentor, teacher, or car pool driver, children in modern society more than ever spend a great deal of time outside their homes with trusted others, time that is unsuper-vised by parents or other family members. And it is in the context of these ongoing relationships that the fundamental trust between an adult and child is all too often incrementally violated in secrecy, thus beginning a relationship that over time becomes ever more confusing and traumatizing for the victim. Kayla describes how insidious the grooming process can be:

And the older I got, the more involved with both judo and Daniel I became. I started traveling all over with him, and he started driving me home from judo at night so my mom wouldn't have to. Sometimes he would even stay the night so that he didn't have to drive home.

When we would travel to tournaments, we would always swim in the pool or wrestle together in one of the hotel rooms. No one found it odd because Daniel was seen as just a big kid . . . just one of us . . . someone who could be trusted.

Once parents and caregivers know to pay attention to telltale changes in a child's or teen's relationship with a specific adult, as well as unexplained shifts in the youth's interests and involvements in daily activities, it becomes more possible to intervene effectively. Knowing both the individual and family factors that have been shown to place a child at greater risk for sexual abuse (see the box on page 14) is also critically important.

It is our hope that the information presented here will be used by families and adults who interact regularly with children to educate children directly about the fact that while "stranger danger" is real, so is the risk of being hurt by an adult well known to them. In fact, simply having this conversation with a child can help forewarn the child in a manner that allows her to both identify and seek assistance quickly should anyone try to touch her inappropriately. This is all the more necessary, as we now know that once sexual abuse begins and goes undiscovered, these children find themselves trapped in an increasingly harrowing situation that they typically have no idea how to escape from. To ring the alarm bells about just how this happens, Kayla reveals precisely what her experience was like the "first time"—when things with Daniel went from touching to sexual assault:

The first time I had sex was not what people always tell you. It wasn't with someone special. It wasn't consensual. But it was something I will never forget. Talking about it is hard. Writing about it for the world is harder. Because what I remember is fragments. It's bits and pieces of a memory I have tried for years to suppress. It is the memories of a child who is so scared that her mind disassociates in order to survive. This is what I remember from that night.

I am young. Maybe I am in middle school. Daniel has come over to spend the night again. It's dark. Mom has gone to bed because she has to work early tomorrow. It's just me and him on my couch. We are watching an action movie on low. Loud enough to make noise but just soft enough so we can hear if people are coming.

I am lying on him. Daniel and I have been "in love" for a year. I know this because we do things together that only people in love do. Most times I don't mind, but sometimes it scares me.

He tells me to lie down. I lie on my stomach, thinking he is going to rub my back like he always does. He turns me over. I look up at him and almost say it. But I'm scared. I don't want to say it and spoil our secret.

He starts touching me over my shirt. I don't mind. I close my eyes and hold on to him, my arms wrapped around his big belly as far as I can. He sits up and starts to pull down my pants.

"Stop," I say.

"Shhh." He pulls harder.

"Daniel, stop. NO." I start to cry. I am scared. He has never done this before.

"Shhhh, baby bird, it's all right. Shhhh." He soothes me with his words as he pulls off my pants.

I am shaking. I am sobbing so hard I cannot breathe. I am frozen.

He pulls down my underwear.

I cry louder.

He puts his hand over my mouth and soothes me.

I am panicking. He lays his body on mine, and I am crushed beneath him. I cannot move. I cannot think. I want to disappear. I want to die. I close my eyes and try to drift away. It's okay. This is love.

One day I will be a bird. I will fly away and I will never come back. Some birds only fly south for the winter, but I will fly forever. My feet will never touch the ground again. **Please God make this be over.**

I cry out. It hurts so much. It hurts so much. It hurts so much. He puts his hand over my mouth and says, "I love you."

Male hippos sometimes kill their young. If a mother and a calf are not careful, a daddy hippo will kill the baby. They are jealous and territorial. **Please God make this be over.**

There is a sun. It's so bright. It's shining on me, and I can feel the warmth on my skin. I am so light and free. It smells like pine trees. The sun fades. **Please God make this be over.**

In my body there is a heart. I will build a fortress around it. I am laying red bricks. Higher and higher they go around my heart. I slather the gray paste between, just like on real buildings. Higher still it goes. My heart is protected forever. Forever. **Please God make this be over.**

Sometimes when I close my eyes real tight and I push my fist into them, I see bright white spots. Some stars. Some stripes. I always think that this is God. He is talking to me. He is saying, it's all right, little lamb. It's all right. I press harder. **Please God make this be over.**

I was a lamb in our preschool Christmas play. I was a lamb first, then the next year I got to be the angel. Maybe if I'm a lamb now, soon I will be an angel. **Please God make this be over.**

Tears are rolling down my face. I can't stop shivering. There is blood on the couch.

"Go get some paper towels and soap, baby bird."

I go to the bathroom. I look in the mirror. I look away. I am so dirty. He washes the cushion and flips it over. The evidence is gone from the ugly brown couch. I wish the evidence was gone from me.

"Come here, bird. Lie down with me." I lie down. He rubs my back. I pretend to fall asleep. I want to rip out my soul.

Do I have a soul? I want to rip out my heart. I want to crawl out of my skin. He moves to the other couch. All night long I count his snores.

2

Keeping the Secret

January 7, 2004 (age 13)

He's pissed at me. I keep messing up, and it's making him angrier and angrier. It doesn't help that I've been so distant lately. Middle school is hard. Making friends is hard, and just dealing with life has been hard. Leading two lives is wearing on me.

"Kayla, go with Fat Boy," he says. I look at Michael and smile weakly. I'm sure he hates being called Fat Boy. We spar, and he goes easy on me. I'm grateful because he is over 50 pounds heavier than me. But apparently this only increases Daniel's rage. The buzzer rings, and I bow to Michael and shake his hand.

"You're going with me now," Daniel says. I freeze. This isn't going to be good. At 5'4" and 106 pounds I am no match for his 6'1" 230-pound frame.

There are times when Daniel is so much fun. He can make me laugh more than anyone in the world. He can joke and tease and tickle. He can own an audience and a room. He can be sweet. But today is not one of those days. Today is the other Daniel. The one that scares me.

The buzzer rings, and we bow to start the round. I try to circle and move to kill time, but he's not having any of it. He grabs me straight away and starts controlling my movements. After all these years and all this training, I am still helpless against him. He puts me on my back hard, and my breath rushes out. I want to cry but know that if I do it will only make it worse. So instead I get angry. I take the anger and I hold on to it.

I get up and go after him. I surprise him and get him off balance with a foot sweep. It's nothing really but enough to really end it for me. I have woken the beast. He slams his hand down my back, jarring my body. By now everyone has stopped to watch. I know it's only a matter of seconds before the pain arrives and I try to think, but thinking doesn't work . . . We take a step, then a second, and on the third he comes across and picks me up. I think as I am in the air that maybe the fall won't be so bad. Maybe it won't hurt so much. But then his feet start coming off the mat too, and I realize what he's going to do. I close my eyes and wait for the impact. We both go in the air, and his 230-pound body comes crashing down on me. But the angle is wrong. My arm has gotten caught and twisted. I feel a pop and a sharp pain and instantly cry out. Something is wrong.

*   *   *

Tears are streaming down my face as I try to sit up.

"Will you stop your goddamned crying," he snarls. "Jesus Christ, you'd think after all these years you'd be a little f***ing tougher."

I swallow hard and bite the inside of my cheek. I'm fine. I'm fine. I'm fine. I am not fine. My arm is throbbing and it feels so heavy. Michael gingerly helps me get to my feet. I cry out a little. I can't help it.

*"Go put a shirt on. I'm going to call your mom and have her meet us at the hospital," Daniel tells me. Putting a shirt on proves difficult. He comes in the women's changing room and helps. He is gentler now. He is changing back into nice Daniel. I can see his breath catch as he pulls off my sweaty top. **Even in pain I am relieved to know that I please him.***

*   *   *

In the car he rubs my leg.

"Next time, just do what you're told and something like this won't happen, bird. If you would only listen to me, you would never have gotten hurt. I don't understand what goes through your head, but you better fucking figure it out. You better start getting your shit together. Stop fucking up."

I nod. I listen. I am a screw-up. I am stupid. I am in so much freaking pain. "Make a fist. You don't want the blood supply to stop. Make a fist."

"But it hurts," I say.

"Make a fucking fist. And don't fucking stop until we get to the hospital. I don't want the blood supply to stop in case it's just muscular."

I look out the window, and tears roll down.

*   *   *

We wait in the waiting room for several hours before they x-ray me. Mom comes and checks me in, but she is on call, so she has to leave again. Daniel says he will stay the night and take me home. I try not to panic. I should be happy. A night with Daniel is rare. But it hurts so much just to hold still and breathe.

I have a broken collarbone, and my humerus is split in two. There's nothing they can do tonight, so Mom will have to bring me tomorrow. They give me a sling and some pain pills. I am grateful for those.

In the car Daniel gives me one and pops two. He looks over at me, worried, and I can tell he is sorry. He doesn't have to say it. I grab his hand.

"I'm okay," I say.

"I know, baby."

"It doesn't even hurt."

"That's my girl. That's my baby bird," he says. I smile and look out the window.

*   *   *

It's 2:00 A.M. by the time we pull into my drive. My younger brother, sister, and my parents are all asleep. We creep in as quiet as we can. By now I am woozy from the pain pill and no food. I don't ask for food, though, because I know it will make him mad. I'm fine.

He takes my hand and leads me to the couch. Inside I am screaming. My arm and collarbone are broken. I am tired. I am weak. I am in so much pain. **Please don't make me screw you. Please. Please. I can't do it tonight. I can't.** On the outside my expression remains blank. I am emotionless. He sits down and pulls me onto his lap.

"I love you," he says.
"I love you too." He kisses me. I kiss back. He pushes me down to the ground in front of him, and I whimper. He pushes more firmly. I close my eyes. I'm fine.

For children like Kayla, victimized sexually during their childhood by adults they know and trust, the encounter and its aftermath described above is nothing out of the ordinary. Obviously not all incidences involve broken bones, but there is always some form of coercion involved as the perpetrator uses the power of his position—as a parent, clergyperson, teacher, or neighbor—to extract sexual favors from the child. As explained in Chapter 1, the perpetrator is often someone the child and family have come to rely on in significant ways, and over time it becomes increasingly difficult for the child to divulge the nature of the relationship and risk losing this benefit.

Using coercion is not the only way that abusers gain a stronger and stronger hold over their victims. Communicating in various ways that these youth will pay a huge toll for disrupting and/or disclosing the relationship, abusers leave them fearful of reprisal, both physical and emotional, if they don't keep the secret. As a result, these children engage in more and more desperate attempts to appease their offenders and normalize the boundary violations that now define their daily lives.

Typical types of threats are listed in the box on page 34. In most cases the abused child will not reveal that she's being threatened in any of these ways, but strong resistance to missing a regularly scheduled interaction with an adult can be a red flag. On page 77, for example, Kayla describes an instance when she stunned her parents with a violent reaction to being told she couldn't attend a team sleepover. Of course there can be many innocuous reasons for a child's not wanting his routine to change.

> If your child strongly resists changing plans or otherwise failing to meet a certain adult's expectations, pay attention. Does this relationship fall outside the bounds of what's normal for adults and children?

A child might not want to miss Little League practice because he knows there are three other pitchers just waiting to be the next starter. A teen might not want to miss a tutoring session because she really wants to raise her GPA and get into the college of her choice. But resistance that includes vehement objections to disappointing the adult in charge may be worth paying attention to. Being abused also

COMMON THREATS FROM PERPETRATORS

To control their victims, child abusers often threaten the child with promises of

- Physical harm
- Loss of support
- Harm to someone in the child's family
- Loss of support to the family
- Getting into trouble
- Being revealed as a "liar" (because the child has purportedly misinterpreted the behavior)

creates deep and complicated confusion in children's minds: Is this normal? What does it mean? Does this person care about me (as most abusers claim)? Is this my fault? Why does this make me feel special sometimes but different and bad at other times?

For those close to a child who is or may be a victim of sexual abuse, it's important to know not only why children don't reveal what's going on but also how this traumatizing experience results in baffling behavior from the children and how the ongoing silence actually perpetuates itself. Victims like Kayla, whose abuse starts when they are quite young, most often adjust to their abuse by learning to first think and then act as if nothing is wrong. Ironically, it is these very accommodations to the abuse that keep the child trapped in the relationship and silent.

Writing in her journal during the period following her first full sexual incident with Daniel, Kayla speaks to the deepening riddle of her changed existence and conflicting self-perceptions:

After that night I first had sex with Daniel, my life changed forever. I felt as if I had made a choice and no matter what I could not go back.

I could not love anyone but Daniel. After all, I needed him. I wanted to be a successful athlete. I wanted to be a star. And I was obsessed with this idea and the idea of him. One was connected to the other. Judo, Daniel. Daniel, judo.

And as his hold on me grew stronger and stronger, my life became more and more a lie. I felt as if I were two people. And that there was no way out . . . and I started to change. Slowly I stopped hanging out with my friends. In the mornings I would go for a run, and then after school I would work out in the school gym and then head straight to judo.

As my athletic career started progressing it seemed as if my social skills stopped working altogether. I would wear sweatpants every day. And I stopped looking people in the eye. I still did well in school and seemed to be okay to the outside world, but on the inside I was in constant torment.

Torn between hating myself and the lies I was living and hating Daniel and wishing I would never see him again. But also needing him and knowing he was my one shot at a life I so longed for.

And loving him despite all of the hate. Well, thinking I loved him anyway. And this is all going on in my head while worrying about what grade I'm going to get on my math quiz.

In order to stay sane I started keeping a journal. I had kept one for a while, but the older I got the more dark and suicidal my writing became. I often wonder how different my life would have been if someone had just read it. Just once . . . and believed what they read.

WHY VICTIMS MAINTAIN THEIR SILENCE

As Kayla describes above, a child who is being abused sexually has to wrestle with confusing contradictions. *Due to the very imbalance of power* that lies at the heart of adult–child relationships, a familiar adult's violation of society's prescribed boundaries leaves the child victim with essentially little choice but to work to maintain an attachment to the very person who is hurting her. These efforts often focus on trying to be "good" to please or appease the abuser. Some children spend a great deal of time doing so, increasing their isolation and widening the distance between themselves and the adults and friends who might offer relief and protection.

Trying to Normalize the Abnormal

Imagine what it must feel like for a young child, whose mental capacity is still in the process of development, to be forced to learn to "preserve a sense of trust in people who are untrustworthy, safety in a situation that is unsafe, . . . and power in a situation of helplessness," as Judy Herman put it so clearly in her pioneering 1992 book, *Trauma and Recovery*. Child sexual abuse flies in the face of everything children have been taught to expect from the adults who care about them. This left Kayla, as it does most victims, in the position of having to learn to act and think as if nothing in her relationship with Daniel was wrong—and to respond to the outer world as if everything was as it should be, even in the face of her ever more difficult daily reality.

It can be impossibly hard to imagine the emotional predicament of the children who must struggle against the awareness that a loved and trusted adult may be hurting them on purpose. As Herman writes in the 1997 revised edition of her seminal book, "the abused child's . . . task is . . . formidable . . . to preserve her *faith* in her parents or other primary caregiver [or another trusted adult, like Kayla's coach, Daniel] she must reject the first and most obvious conclusion that something is terribly wrong with [the adult]." Herman called the dilemma of having to hold contradictory and unacceptable realities in mind and survive "doublethink," borrowing a famous term from George Orwell. This phenomenon forces abused children to deny and dissociate from reality because they simply can't reconcile these disturbing contradictions. The inability to do so is one reason abused children remain silent, and the mental effort involved in turn exacts a high toll (see the box on page 37).

Abused children use multiple psychological techniques to try to transform the reality of their abuse into something more acceptable and manageable, from suppressing memories of specific incidents to minimizing the betrayal, to rationalizing what's going on, and to completely denying that anything out of the ordinary is happening. It's important to understand that children often don't even realize they're using these mental machinations, but the profound confusion involved in trying to make sense of the inexplicable violation they are suffering leaves most children feeling unable to speak about their abuse. A clear example of this is the case of clergy abuse. Before the Boston scandal depicted in the movie *Spotlight* became public, as related in a 2002 *Boston Globe Special Report*, priests were seen as sacrosanct keepers of morality and spiritual guides for parishioners, creating an impossible situation for victims of their abuse. Disclosure by these victims was put off for extended periods of time as the children involved questioned their own grasp of reality and tried to reconcile the priests' holy image with their thoroughly unholy behavior.

THE HIGH COST OF DOUBLETHINK

The "doublethink" of having to deal with the reality of a trusted, possibly beloved, adult hurting them leaves abused children in a state where they may be prone to thinking and behaving in a disjointed fashion. Your child may, in fact, be only intermittently aware of the reality of the abuse. She may seem to be daydreaming or "out of it" and can display unexplained gaps in memory, focus, and functioning. This phenomenon has become equated, in modern psychiatric parlance, with symptoms of dissociation— symptoms that are frequently part of the picture that we see with children subjected to chronic sexual abuse.

Parents we see often report that, looking back, they remember that their child began acting "differently" at a specific point in time, but regrettably did not understand the possible significance of these observed changes in behavior. The symptoms we most frequently hear in this regard that parents noticed include

- Decline in focus: "I would have to remind her ten times to get something done."
- Forgetfulness: "She starting losing things wherever she went; that was not her."
- Complaints from school: "The teacher said she 'daydreamed' and seemed sad."
- Unexplained exhaustion: "She complained of insomnia and always was tired."
- Daydreaming: "She always seemed in her own head . . . somewhere else."

If you see these signs, what should you do?

While these signs alone *do not* indicate that a child is being hurt by someone, they are noteworthy if they appear suddenly and in combination, and especially if you have any concerns about an intensifying relationship between your child and an adult in his or her life, and then may warrant a trip to the pediatrician. Unless you have suspicions about a *specific* relationship, however, don't go on a "fishing expedition" with the child about random adults in his life or suggest to the pediatrician that your child might be the victim of abuse. Simply describe the symptoms you're observing. Your pediatrician should then try to narrow down possible causes of disjointed behavior and thinking, which can include asking your child directly, *often while you are out of the room,* if anything is bothering him that he is keeping to himself or is afraid to talk about. Sometimes the expertise and objectivity of the pediatrician can elicit information from a child that he has been unable or unwilling to share with a parent. (How you can talk with your child about specific suspicions is covered at length in Chapter 3.)

Trying to Reconcile "Good" and "Bad"

The destructive impact of CSA on its victims includes not just disruptions in how the abused children come to perceive the world; it also extends to how they begin to see themselves. As a child tries to find some meaning that would justify the reality of the abuse that she cannot entirely avoid, she will often begin to create what Judy Herman termed in 1992 a *double-self*, believing she is bad as a way of preserving the wish that the person hurting her—whether a parent, coach, or clergyperson—is still somehow good and just. This belief in their own "inner badness" frequently keeps children locked in silence as well. Especially when the abuse continues for many years, victims believe that their badness is borne out both by being selected by the perpetrator in the first place and then by their ongoing *cooperation* in maintaining the silence and secrecy. Naturally this rationale brings with it crushing, and silencing, guilt and shame. Feeling a grave sense of self-blame and shame is the number one issue we, as clinicians, deal with when treating these children, and a key focus of treatment needs to always be on helping them begin to understand that they are in no way responsible for the perpetrator's actions.

The phenomenon of trying to deny aspects of reality and reassign responsibility to preserve an abusive relationship can be seen clearly in Kayla's writings from the age of 13, shortly after the sexual abuse begins in earnest, as she struggles to convince herself that the relationship with Daniel can survive:

September 1, 2003 (age 13)

Dear God,

Hi. How are you? I'm fine. Thank you for helping me win all those tournaments. It gave me confidence in myself and I believe I can beat all of those girls. Thank you.

God, age doesn't matter, right? Because it's illegal now but not forever. I really like him and obviously he must like me a little, right God? That's what people do when they like you.

But God is he just using me? Because I really think I love him. Am I too young to be experiencing this or not? Does age even matter? He says not to worry, but I do, very much so. I don't want him to get caught and I don't want to get in trouble.

Is our relationship more than just, you know, . . . Physical? Or does he just use me? I hope not. Well, I do as he says and not worry about it, or at least not talk to anyone about it but you God.

Love Always,
Kayla

Struggling to Distinguish Right from Wrong

Kayla's questions to God illustrate the dilemma that abused children face due to their developmental age: Their grasp of what's right and wrong is a work in progress. Where sexual abuse involves physical pain (from penetration and other invasive sexual violations), the child certainly knows she is being hurt. The question in her mind, then, is why: Why would someone who is supposed to be in a protective role (an authoritative adult) do the opposite? Children will wrestle with this question of what "authority" actually means, only gradually maturing enough to develop an understanding of what they should expect from adults in care-giving roles.

But even more confusing is their immature understanding of sex and its role in life. By preschool most children have begun to explore their own bodies purposefully, by touching themselves, and can identify their own gender. At this time it is often wise to begin to talk with your children about not letting anyone, not even family members or other people they trust, touch them in a way that feels uncomfortable. At this age, however, children have no concept of what "sex" actually is and cannot answer questions about procreation. By ages 6–10 children typically become more inquisitive about topics such as pregnancy and the specifics of sex and where babies come from. During this time period, however, children also remain very dependent on adults to distinguish "right" from "wrong," are expected to obey adults, and often don't have a sufficient understanding of sexual rules and mores to know clearly when an adult is beginning to groom them or engage in inappropriate touching. As children mature sexually during puberty, they start to get a clearer idea about their own physical boundaries and what types of touching are inappropriate and unwelcome; this is why adolescence is a period when teens may disclose abuse that has been going on since earlier in childhood. Perpetrators often take advantage of both a younger child's naiveté and their own authority to do harm.

In the preceding journal entry we can see that Kayla is beginning to ask many more questions about what was right and what was wrong about her relationship with Daniel. Unfortunately, the fact that the abuse remained a secret meant she had no source of reliable answers, and her mounting confusion and despair was taking an increasing toll on her sense of self-esteem and self-worth:

September 7, 2003 (age 13)

Dear God,

Hi. How are you? I'm doing okay. I need to talk to someone about my relationship with . . . And, well, I can't tell anyone except you because if I do I'll get him in trouble and I'll be in trouble too he says.

So I hope you understand now that I'm too far in to back out now. I really like him and I feel the urge to be around him all the time. It's funny, but I think he needs me too. He makes me feel special but also dirty. When I see him and think about what we share, I have so much inside me I don't know what to do with it. I feel loved, but I also hate myself.

Please, God, don't let us get caught. It would ruin everything, and I don't want that to happen. I also get jealous and hate him when I see him with other girls, God. Does this mean we're together or not? I feel like I'm already so attached, and that's not good. So I don't know. I lie in bed at night and think about everything and wonder if he's thinking about me too.

God. I dream about him and the Olympics and someday being the person everyone wants me to be, God. God, please don't let us get caught.

And thank you for your help at the last tournament. I was happy with 4th. Even if he wasn't.

Love Always,
Kayla

Weighed Down by Self-Blame and Shame

Again, when children start being abused at a young age as they typically are (remember the median age for CSA to begin is 9), they commonly lack an understanding of personal boundaries and societal norms and therefore often don't initially fully recognize that what the perpetrator is doing is considered wrong. This innocence is further reinforced by the perpetrator, who has worked to gradually desensitize the child to physical touching, disguising it first as a game and then gradually progressing to sexualized contact. Unfortunately, when child victims over time inevitably become more aware that what is happening *is* abuse, they already have come to see themselves as coconspirators and deserving of the abuse in some fashion, especially if the relationship has continued for a prolonged period and they have been unable to surmount the barriers to disclosure. By owning some of this *badness,* they make the powerful and important adult involved less reprehensible and the attachment can, at least temporarily, be preserved.

What we also know is that the more essential and central the abusive adult is in a child's life and to her well-being, the more willing the child can be to either deny the reality of the wrongdoing altogether or take "the evil of the abuser into herself," as Judith Herman writes. This leads to the lowered self-esteem, the inability to regulate both mood and attention, and problems with trust that we see in sexually abused children when they come to us for professional help. Another complication is that when we finally do see these children, they have frequently spent months or years in the grip of the perpetrator, camouflaging the trauma to preserve the status quo, fighting to appear efficient, successful, competent, and unharmed to the outside world while continuing to suffer within. The reality of her abuse and mounting desperation about secrecy are captured by Kayla again at age 13 when she writes in her journal about fears that she might be pregnant:

October 1, 2003 (age 13)

Dear God,

Hi. How are you? I'm fine. I'm feeling a little depressed though. I have to talk to you about something. God am I—? Please don't let me be. I will die if I am. God I would not be able to take it if I was. I would be crushed. God, please don't let that be the case.

God, I'm sorry for all the bad things I've done. I wish my life were not so complicated, like Kristy's or Heather's. I don't know how to feel. I am not letting him do that again.

Love always,
Kayla
Amen.

Becoming More and More Dependent on— and Isolated by—the Abuser

CSA perpetrators not only take advantage of their ability to offer some practical benefit (such as coaching or tutoring) to their victims but commonly also offer a desirable sense of connection. This may be particularly alluring to children who have been targeted because they are in fact already lonely or isolated, but even for those like Kayla who are not, an increasing sense of emotional connection can cement the victim's loyalty and secure her silence. Victims tell us that their abuser was often their most intimate confidant. Children shared with them their life problems, dreams and aspirations, and struggles in relationships, including those with their family. The abuser became the primary source of emotional support. This is a difficult benefit for many children to risk losing. We are told that a sudden withdrawal of this support when the abuse is revealed, together with doubts about whom to turn to now, leads them to experience intolerable loneliness and despair in the aftermath of disclosure. This is part of a phenomenon that bewilders the loved ones of the victim: just when they are finally "saved" abused children and teens often descend into helplessness, despair, and declining overall functioning (all discussed in more depth in Chapter 5). It must be added here that for a percentage of children and teens who are victimized by sexual abuse, even when their perpetrator is initially a family member or trusted adult, they remain silent simply from a fear of retaliation from both the perpetrator and the other adults they rely on, and report never having experienced even a second of comfort or emotional support from their abuser. Put simply, it is the power differential and unknown consequences of breaking their silence that keep many trapped in the abusive relationship for prolonged periods of time.

As the perpetrator works behind the scenes to communicate, both overtly and indirectly, that the consequences of disclosure or discovery will be catastrophic, the victimized child becomes increasingly isolated within the abuser's sphere of control. In the descriptions of what happened in her relationships with her family, closest friends, and teammates, Kayla's writings from this period indicate her awareness of the schism developing with significant others, and yet her focus remains on preserving what she needs and depends on most—the all-consuming relationship with Daniel, who has gradually become the center of her universe and who she believes is key to her ongoing athletic success. One of Kayla's early journal entries from this time indicates this tension and speaks to her increasing confusion about how to think about the relationship with Daniel:

April 12, 2004 (age 13)

Dear God,

It's very late, so I will keep it short and simple. Sorry to have not written you in so long. I'm trying to keep up, but at night when I crawl into bed I'm too exhausted to write you.

I will try harder. Mom thinks I have a crush on Daniel, but I don't. He's more of a really really good friend. The only one I can talk to. The thought of people getting the wrong idea about us sickens me.

God forgive them.

Love Always,
Kayla

Wrestling with What "Love" Means

As with their understanding of "sex," children's understanding of what "love" means evolves and changes as they mature. Preschool children generally use the word "love" to describe how they feel about close relatives such as parents and grandparents and to describe how these relatives feel about them. This family-centered definition of love expands when children enter school, and it's not unusual for children ages 6–10 to talk about having a "boyfriend" or "girlfriend" of the same age and to describe these relationships in a loving fashion. With the onset of puberty, however, the concept of "love" expands even further to include not only age-mates but also older persons whom the adolescent may look up to, depend on, or have a crush on. We've all seen teens revere adult rock stars, athletes, and movie stars, and we may even remember from our own experience at this age that this adulation often involves fantasizing about sharing physical intimacy with these individuals. The same types of crushes can easily extend during adolescence to beloved teachers, coaches, and others whom the child knows personally, leaving them vulnerable to inappropriate sexual advances by these adults.

> ## HOW DIFFERENT RELATIONSHIPS CREATE SILENT VICTIMS
>
> Depending on who the perpetrator is, children may actually feel that they are "in love" with that person, particularly before they are old enough to be *fully aware* that the relationship violates societal norms. In other instances, as in cases of clergy or educator abuse, the targeted child more often feels admiration for or deference to the perpetrator, rather than love, and keeps silent out of respect for and fear of the perpetrator's authority. And in the 10–25% of cases where there is no preexisting relationship to the abuser, victims may remain silent because they fear a reprisal and loss of privacy. In all these instances, even when children believe they are in love with their perpetrators, remember that this is nonetheless an abuse of power situation in which elements of force and fear are universally present to some degree.

Thus feeling love for someone, or feeling loved by him, can underlie sexual boundary violations that occur during the teen years when the adolescent understands the concept of inappropriate sexual touching but has come eventually to believe that a particular adult's love for her, as in Kayla's case, overrides these rules. Once "in love" with the older adult, the teen, at least initially, can see the sexual contact as consensual, even though the he or she is under the age of consent and the touching remains illegal and constitutes abuse in the eyes of the law. (The age of consent and other legal issues are discussed in Chapter 4.)

This issue of a child "loving" an adult who sexually abuses him or her is that much more complicated in cases of incest, where a blood relationship between perpetrator and victim exists. The great majority of all cases of child sexual abuse involve a perpetrator known to the child, and approximately one-third of these involve family members.

Trying to Protect the Family

The push to maintain the status quo and stay silent is particularly strong when the abuser is a family member. In these cases disclosing or being discovered carries the added threat of destroying the entire family. Often the abuser threatens the child with this possibility: If she tells, her family will no longer be together and she will be compelled to live in another home. Or, let's say the abuser is an uncle; he might tell his niece that disclosing the abuse will hurt her mother, who is his sister, and she'll never forgive the child for making this accusation. Or if the abuser is her father, he'll say he'd end up in prison, and the family would have no means of support. The real life impact of disclosing incest can thus be great, and the child questions whether anything, even his own safety, is worth "blowing up" the family.

Getting the Message That the Truth Is Unwelcome

In situations of incest it can be very difficult for the nonoffending parent to accept that someone in her own family, a father or brother in most cases, actually has sexually victimized a child relative. But even when the perpetrator is not related, but was a close friend or had some connection to the child's family, finding out about the abuse can be particularly painful for parents and other family members to accept. Knowing that their revelations will emotionally hurt others whom they love and rely on can be a strong deterrent for child victims. Children can anticipate this outcome and hesitate further, prolonging the abuse. In our experience with cases of incest, the child is typically well aware that her revelation of what has been happening to her will likely be unwelcome to some, if not all, members of her family. Mothers who learn that their husbands or other children have been sexually abusing a younger child describe the devastating moment when they fully realized that acceptance of the "truth" of the disclosure will forever shatter the family life they thought they had. This realization can lead to myriad painful and conflicting responses, from questioning the veracity of the revelations to feeling like an "utter failure" as a parent. This attachment of one or more of the parents to the abuser makes breaking the silence that much more difficult and in this way can prolong the trauma.

In the words of one mother on learning that her husband had abused their daughter for several years:

> "I still feel dreadful that at first I did not know whether to believe Christina; what she was telling me seemed unimaginable, something you see on TV or in the movies. I always thought that I knew exactly what my kids were thinking and feeling, especially Christina. But then I quickly realized that it must be true;

why would Christina make something like that up, and she was clearly so scared and then it all made sense to me: the unexplained crying and nightmares and how she had asked to get a lock put on her bedroom door that she said was to keep her siblings out. And then I thought, "What will happen to us?" . . . I had no money and no family and was way too embarrassed to tell my friends . . . and then I started to think that this happened because I was not a good enough wife, but then I kept coming back to that there is just no excuse for what he did . . . having sex with our daughter. Looking back, maybe the hardest part was to accept just how wrong I had been about Robert and how at times I felt like I could literally kill the man I married and had my children with. It was a nightmare that I never thought could happen to me and my family."

Suggestions that your child is being abused sexually are shocking enough; the idea that the perpetrator is someone who is loved and trusted by the family makes it even harder to hear with an open mind. As we'll discuss throughout this book, children often try to broach the subject, sometimes indirectly, and then clam up when greeted with hesitation and/or disbelief by a parent or other adult. This is why it's so crucial to try to hear such messages without judging the child. It's why it is so critical to see the signs that a child may be trying to reveal abuse.

THE MYTH THAT "I WOULD KNOW IF SOMETHING WAS WRONG!"

As you can see, children who are suffering sexual abuse go through agonizing mental and emotional gyrations in an attempt to understand what's happening to them and try to soothe themselves. The signs of their internal distress are often disproportionately subtle, so it's not surprising that adults often don't see those signs or misinterpret them. Unfortunately, because sexual abuse is such a horrible transgression, we assume that we *would somehow know* if a child close to us was being hurt. More important, we also assume that the child *would try to tell us* immediately if something bad was happening to him. Parents who are devoted to loving and caring for their children are sure that they're so attuned to their child that he would tell them of any abuse or they would just see it. Teachers who shepherd their students safely through the school day assume they would notice if a child was suffering.

Time and again, adults who have learned that their child has been sexually abused say that what they continue to struggle with most of all is that they *should have known what was happening to their child and been able to stop it.* With that deep regret comes overwhelming guilt and self-blame, typically alternating with blame of the perpetrator. But the fact is that children are not inclined to tell a trusted adult or peer that they need help with sexual abuse as they might be in cases of physical or emotional pain. In these cases the victim often shares a complex and complicated relationship with the perpetrator (see the box on page 44) and quickly becomes caught in a web of shame, secrecy, and emotional dependence we've already described. If the child cannot tell others quickly, when the abuse first begins, she may remain silent for years, and even frequently into adulthood. The fact that children often *can't* extricate themselves from these relationships makes education about the existence and specifics of CSA vastly important to identifying and interrupting this process earlier.

AN IMPORTANT REALITY CHECK

A major goal of this book is to decrease the incidence of CSA by increasing the awareness of it and hopefully reducing its prevalence through education, so we urge all adults to take those sneaking feelings, nagging suspicions, and repeated observations about possible abuse of a child in their care very seriously. *But* that does not mean we advocate fishing expeditions, as noted earlier—such as planting suggestions in a child's mind, which has been found to produce false accusations that in themselves are harmful, or jumping to conclusions impulsively at the first hint that something might be wrong. It's important to bear in mind that it will likely be impossible to ever fully eradicate the sexual abuse of children. And even when forewarned with up-to-date information, parents and caregivers are always vulnerable to missing a trail that the abuser is trying mightily to cover up. What's the take-home message here? Keep your eyes open, think rationally, and follow up when your concerns are strong and persistent. How to talk to a child to elicit a disclosure of any abuse that's occurring and how to deal with the authorities in charge of investigating cases of abuse are covered in Chapters 3 and 4.

HOW LONG DO CHILDREN WAIT
TO BREAK THEIR SILENCE?

The fact that children often wait years before feeling able to disclose their abuse does not mean they don't try to extricate themselves during their period of silence. Over time many of them hit a point where they actively think about ending the abusive relationship and wonder if they can do so without disclosing. By this time both the relationship itself and the related secrecy are typically causing them profound distress, and the perils of maintaining the status quo are ever present. This can be seen in Kayla's diary entry on October 20, as she talks about her confusion and the experience of wondering if she in fact has the strength to say "no" to Daniel, as she worries about a potential pregnancy:

October 20, 2003 (age 13)

Dear God,

    Hi. It's just me again. I know I just wrote you, but I need to talk to you. I know I'm not now, I can't be. There's no way to be sure, so I'm still worried, but not as worried as I was. God, please give me the strength to say no.

    I don't want to do this anymore. Please. I will be strong and say no, or at least try. Please help me. Thank you.

    Love always,
    Kayla

    While it's difficult for many reasons to arrive at a precise estimate of how many children disclose their abuse while it's occurring, most studies consistently suggest that *less than half* of children who are being sexually abused report this abuse during childhood, and for those who do report it, there is a significant delay between when the abuse starts and when victims disclose. Research in the area of CSA consistently reveals that many victims live with their secret until directly asked as an adult about any past sexual abuse they had endured. While for abuse with a physical component there may be signs such as a bruise, scratch, or broken bone, children who are sexually abused most typically show no outward signs or symptoms of what they are privately suffering through. Inherent in the very secretive nature of CSA is the reality that it still all too often falls to the child alone to figure out how, when, and to whom she can most safely disclose her abuse.

So what more do we know about the rate and timing of disclosures of CSA and other forms of childhood abuse? Here are some highlights:

- Based on a 2005 review of the literature by London and colleagues, only about 34% of child sexual abuse victims disclosed their abuse either immediately or soon after it started, with most victims of CSA waiting from many months to many years to reveal their abuse.

- Despite greater awareness by the public, more recent studies, such as the one done by Catherine Townsend and colleagues in 2016, indicate that the rates of disclosure have remained at less than one-third.

- Even when there's corroborative evidence—including physical evidence or confessions from the abuser and/or evidence provided by bystander witness—researchers Lyon and colleagues continue to find that up to 43% of children remain unwilling or unable to disclose their sexual abuse.

Given that a majority of children who are abused sexually stay silent for months or even years, it's important for parents, caregivers, and educators to know the emotional and behavioral symptoms that may well signal that a child is being abused.

> Greater knowledge of the signs of child sexual abuse → more effective intervention.

THE HIGH PRICE OF SILENCE

The reluctance to disclose, regardless of reason, leads to multi-incident abuse for many victims, as Jim Henry found in a 1997 study, in which 53% of the 90 children in his sample group were abused more than five times before disclosing their abuse. Moreover, the average age of disclosure was 13 in this study, while the mean age for the onset of abuse was 11—a full 2-year gap between the time when the abuse started and when the abuse was revealed. Mary Paine reported similar findings in 2002. And a 2007 study by Hershkowitz and colleagues found that 92% of the victims of more severe CSA offenses and 86% of multiple-incident abuse delayed their disclosures, indicating again just how hard it becomes for victims to disclose sexual abuse once the cycle begins and endures over time.

We now know that children like Kayla, who are subjected to prolonged sexual abuse, begin to experience recognizable patterns of psychological and behavioral symptoms. These symptoms are present both during childhood as the abuse is occurring and potentially into adulthood.

Harm That Often Continues after the Abuse Has Ended

These symptoms often begin as what is technically called an "acute stress response" to the initiation of the abuse and include difficulties with sleeping, concentrating, eating, and interacting with others. Then symptoms can increase and worsen as the abuse continues to include identity confusion and diffuse emotional distress, difficulties described poignantly by Kayla in the journal entries during the years of her victimization. What's important for parents and other adults to understand is that silence does not mean the child isn't suffering. The gradual alterations in their belief system and the emotional adjustment and adaptations to daily life that the abuse forces them to make can take an enormous toll. The longer a child remains in a state of having to adapt and survive in a sexually abusive situation, the more challenging it can be for the child to recover from the multiple impacts of the abuse.

> Never interpret silence from a child as an indication that nothing is wrong and the child is fine. In assessing whether something is wrong with a child, notice whether there is a sudden change in behavior. For instance, sudden secretiveness, isolation, or more than usual irritability can indicate that there is an underlying problem worth further exploration. Children can be silent and brooding, but their silence does not necessarily mean there is nothing wrong.

In fact, when a child is being victimized sexually, whether or not the child discloses the abuse or exhibits symptoms at the time, there is a great likelihood that the child's emotions, beliefs, and behaviors are being altered in some way by the traumatic experience. Not only are they being altered but, according to an early authority in the field of childhood trauma, Dr. Lenore Terr, in 2003, these effects "appear to last for long periods of life, no matter what diagnosis the patient eventually receives." Terr found at least four characteristics related to chronic childhood trauma:

- Visualized or otherwise repeatedly perceived memories of the traumatic event (such as having repeated nightmares about being hurt).
- Repetitive behaviors connected to the initial trauma (flirting with men without being attracted to them, for example).
- Trauma-specific fears (such as thinking that any man who likes you will try to molest you).
- Changed attitudes about people, life, and the future (thinking that you are destined to lose at anything you try and the like).

What is important to note about this symptom picture is that it describes elements of posttraumatic stress disorder (PTSD), a psychiatric disorder in which a known trauma has occurred and the individual who has been "traumatized" is experiencing symptoms, including those identified by Terr, that persist for more than a month following the trauma (see the box on page 52).

Silence May Deny Children the Treatment They Need

Research conducted by Beth Molnar and associates in 2001 on mental health problems following abuse showed that these problems increased with the severity and duration of the abuse and when the perpetrator was not a stranger. Unfortunately, the diagnostic criteria (see the box on page 52) require a known trauma to make a diagnosis of PTSD. Silence therefore can rob an abused child of the very treatment needed to address the effects of the trauma.

Children who exhibit the symptoms of stress from a trauma when there has been no disclosure of CSA often receive partial diagnoses, leading to only partial treatment of their problems. For example, a child with trouble concentrating and avoiding school might be given a diagnosis of an anxiety disorder and encouraged to gradually reenter the classroom. If in

> Without a diagnosis of PTSD, a child is less likely to receive the most effective treatment to address the trauma of sexual abuse.

POSTTRAUMATIC STRESS DISORDER

Mental health professionals use the criteria in the American Psychiatric Association's 2013 *Diagnostic and Statistical Manual of Mental Disorders* (DSM-5) to diagnose disorders such as PTSD. Essentially, PTSD is characterized by five key features:

1. The person has been exposed to, has witnessed, or has learned about—if a close relative or friend is involved—a traumatic event that involves death, threatened death, actual or threatened serious injury, or actual or threatened sexual violence.

2. The person relives the traumatic event(s), with recurring memories at any time, often feeling the same fear and horror as when the event took place. These reexperienced symptoms could include:
   - Nightmares of the abuse.
   - Flashbacks (feeling like you're going through the event again).
   - Acute emotional distress in response to triggers—seeing, hearing, or smelling something that causes you to relive the event, such as news reports of abuse by coaches, seeing an accident, or hearing a car backfire.

3. The person avoids situations or people that trigger memories of the traumatic event or refrains from talking or thinking about the event:
   - Avoiding crowds, because they feel dangerous.
   - Avoiding driving if abuse repeatedly occurred in a car.
   - Avoiding watching movies about earthquakes if you were in an earthquake.
   - Staying very busy or avoiding seeking help because it prevents having to think or talk about the event.

4. The person's beliefs and feelings related to the trauma change in a negative way:
   - Having unjustified guilt, related to the trauma, that leads you to blame yourself for problems in other relationships.
   - Forgetting about parts of the traumatic event or not being able to talk about it.
   - Thinking the world is completely dangerous, and no one can be trusted.

5. The person feels keyed up in the presence of trauma-related cues—jittery or always alert and on the lookout for danger or suddenly angry or irritable (also called hyperarousal). These symptoms could include:
   - Having a hard time falling and then staying asleep.
   - Having trouble concentrating.
   - Being startled by a loud noise or surprise.
   - Wanting to have your back to a wall in a restaurant or waiting room.

fact the child's avoidance is tied to an abusive relationship within the school setting, she will most often remain in a state of stress and seemingly not respond to the prescribed gold-standard interventions for anxiety problems. This situation highlights how critical it is for us to respond to small signs of distress in our children, particularly if these persist with first-line treatments, and to remain vigilant and curious about the relationships in their lives (more on this problem in Chapter 3).

The danger of not noticing or not responding is that the psychological damage only worsens with time when the symptoms aren't addressed. Chapter 5 goes into detail on the long-term effects of child sexual abuse, and Chapter 6 describes professional help for short- and long-term symptoms. The box below gives a brief overview.

We see evidence of the far-reaching impact of sexual abuse all the time at McLean Hospital. Of the children and teens admitted to our programs, we consistently find that 30–50% have had one or more childhood experiences involving maltreatment and/or trauma. Many

---

LASTING EFFECTS OF CHILD SEXUAL ABUSE

According to the National Center for PTSD (U.S. Department of Veterans Affairs), common mental, emotional, and behavioral problems that can accompany PTSD over the long haul for victims of all types of abuse include:

- Difficulties with anger
- Problems with substance abuse
- Depression
- Self-harming behaviors

There is also a higher rate of medical difficulties found in victims of sexual abuse, including

- Chronic pain
- Respiratory problems
- Headaches
- Panic attacks
- Chronic insomnia
- Gastrointestinal problems
- Urinary tract problems and infections

also have problems with substance abuse and engage in other high-risk behaviors, including self-harm, and a majority trace these difficulties back to the time of their initial abuse. We cannot say it often enough or strongly enough: The cycle of emotional pain associated with sexual abuse, and its impact on many areas of a child's functioning, makes it essential that everyone working with children become educated about the signs that a child is distressed and know how to ask, in a nondirective manner, what might be happening with any child who is showing those signs. The bleeding of distress from sexual abuse into multiple areas of life is a common and unfortunate occurrence described poignantly by Kayla in another of her journal entries:

March 1, 2004 (age 13)

Dear God,

Hi. God, I feel so low and down right now. I did horrible at judo tonight. I have a B in science. But I only have 24 days until Estonia. I feel weak, and my energy is depleted, and I have an eating problem . . . I eat too much. It's like a game I play with my mind: let's see if I'm good enough to sneak food without anyone noticing. I hate the game, but I almost never lose. And I can't stop.

God, please help me. I like to make myself look cooler and I need to stop. My head is swollen, and he needs to deflate me real quickly and I feel like I brag and whine and I'm an attention-seeking bad person.

I don't want to be a bad person anymore. I don't want to start hating judo . . . I can't hate judo. Think of all the people I would disappoint. I love judo.

I feel like I'm sinking deeper and deeper and I can't get back out please help me please. Thank you.

Love Always,
Kayla

In the next chapter we delve into some specifics about what we as caregivers, parents, and friends can do to help detect a situation like Kayla's as early as possible and how to respond sensitively and effectively. Kayla's abuse continued uninterrupted for more than 4 years, as did her confusion about the meaning of the relationship with Daniel: Were they a couple? Was this love? Was this wrong? Kayla continued rising as a judo star, relying only on her journal in a private attempt to sort out the myriad conflicting feelings she harbored for the man whom her family had trusted to be her coach and mentor:

April 7, 2004 (age 13)

Dear God,

Hi. How are you? I'm okay. I'm really mad at Daniel, though.

He gets mad at me because I don't show up to judo, which is usually because no one can take me or I didn't clean my room.

He doesn't come to judo because he's too busy doing something with Ella [Daniel's girlfriend], whatever that may be. And you know if he's even cleaning his house he shouldn't do that during judo time—clean it before.

And he does all this on his own accord! He's a total asshole. Sorry to use such inappropriate language but . . . I'm so angry I can't stand it.

And you know what else is bothering me? I feel sick about my weight. Please help me get it down quick before I can't make weight. Please God just let me make 48 kg for a couple more times please! If I ever miss weight he'll kill me.

Love Always,
Kayla

May 9, 2004 (age 13)

Dear God,

Hi. How are you? I'm a little worried. You know about me and . . . I want to be around him all the time. I wish that he and I could be together without secret but it will never be that way.

My parents would kill me if they knew what we're doing. God please don't let me be . . . I will wait until the end of this month before I say anything.

Please God I'm so sorry for everything I've done and I'm sorry for my sinful ways.

I love you.

Love Always,
Kayla

As is so often true for the victims of sexual abuse, things in Kayla's life intensified as her parents wondered about what was going on in her relationship with Daniel and how to deal with what they suspected without getting any confirmation of their fears from Kayla. For her part, Kayla vehemently rejected their initial worries and denied accusations her mother made after surreptitiously reading several of Kayla's journal entries. This is typically the phase of abuse when a child begins to know that the relationship she is in is wrong somehow, and yet remains very unsure about how to think about it or what to do. Looking back, Kayla says that at that time *"I was EXTREMELY confused, but I was also scared and smart enough to know I could no longer use my journal as an outlet. I would need to be more careful."* Her mother describes to Kayla how her claim that nothing was wrong was so convincing when questioned about the journal entries:

> "When you started showing interest in boys, I was relieved. I was glad you seemed to be fitting into high school even though you were so emotional—everyone told us that was normal. Also, this entry is around the time you became angry with us. You went to live with Mimi. You and I had a really big fight, and we just felt you needed to be out of the house. It was a very tumultuous time. We were thrown off because it seemed to be us you hated, and we were told that was normal teenage angst.
>
> "You must have been extremely adamant. You had a boyfriend and seemed very convincing, so I believed you.

Kayla's words from this period vividly capture the psychological process by which the child clings desperately, albeit with increasing uncertainty, to the view that maybe everything in her life is as it should be—a view that frequently leaves the child increasingly at odds with family members and others who are becoming more and more concerned:

May 31, 2004 (age 13)

Dear God,

Mom questioned me like crazy. She read some of what I write to you. I thought this was the one place I could talk without anyone knowing, but I was wrong. She (thinks she) knows everything. She's officially insane.

I guess a lot of people think that, though. It sickens my stomach.

He's like my best friend, I care about him more than anyone, but the thought of him or any sexual thought of him is just unnatural. He is so much older, and let's face it, he's irresponsible and a drunk. He really doesn't have any qualities I'm looking for in a man.

My stomach aches at every thought of him. I can't have fun with him anymore, and I'm sad. He really is my best friend. He's the only person I willingly tell anything.

I will never be a kid. I cry all the time now.

Sometimes because of Mom. Sometimes because of Daniel. Sometimes because of Dad. Sometimes because of my judo. Sometimes because I didn't get to go to the Olympic trials.

And now my mom thinks I may not be a virgin because I wrote something and she asks if I'm being touched by Daniel, which I told her is insane.

So many things to cry about, God. And yet I try hard not to. This is becoming overwhelming.

Trying to find a way out floods my mind more and more every day.

God, please let this end soon.

Love Always,
Kayla

3

The Tipping Point
BREAKING THE SILENCE

By the fall of 2004, things in my life have really escalated out of control. My (step)father no longer wants me to go to judo, and my mother, whom I have fought hard to convince that everything is okay with Daniel, refuses to let my dad keep me out of judo, saying I'm her daughter and that I have a real chance at being an Olympian.

Because things in the house are so tense and I am fighting nonstop with both my mom and stepdad, I go to stay with my grandparents for a period of time. I'm becoming more and more isolated and desperate, and it is around this time that Brian, the friend whom I will eventually disclose to, starts training at our club, and more and more we begin to develop a strong friendship. After a short time-out with my grandparents, I move back home and once again fight constantly with my parents.

Looking back through my journal entries from this period, I clearly remember having so much hate toward my family, and resented any effort to supervise or control my time with Daniel. There is an entire page in one journal where I just write "I hate my mom. I hate my mom" . . . over and over and over again. And then there are entries like this one, where it is so sad looking back at the turmoil and distress I had lived with and the toll the abuse took on me and everyone around me:

November 7, 2004 (age 14)

Dear God,

Hey, it's me. I'm writing because I hate my mom. She's a bitch and I fucking hate her. She's always on my ass and she has no sympathy for me, so I'm not going to have any for her.

I fucking hate her so much I just wish she'd leave me alone, god.

Please just make everything better. Please God. I hate her and I hate living here.

Please God take me away from here.

Love Always,
Kayla

As discussed in Chapter 2, a child's reluctance to disclose sexual abuse is a complex phenomenon. Many factors can keep children from speaking up. The most common reasons we've heard from children who have been sexually abused are

1. Fearing the consequences to themselves and their family, particularly in instances of incest.
2. Feeling they were to blame for being picked by the perpetrator or continuing to "participate" in the abuse.
3. Lacking understanding at the time the abuse started that it was wrong.
4. Feeling no one would believe them if they disclosed and, if they did, they would be blamed.
5. Fearing loss of a special relationship with the perpetrator.

As we've explained when discussing grooming behavior (Chapter 1) and the common reasons abused children don't disclose (Chapter 2), disclosure is often *intentionally* made more difficult by the abuser, who actively tries to frighten his victim, directly and/or by targeting the child's bond with her mother or another important family member, so that the child ends up believing these adults may not protect him or her, may be angry, or might not even believe the disclosure. Heather Bacon highlighted these dynamics when she wrote in 2001 about her work with 121 victims of CSA in the Cleveland area, who had been taken into protective services and later returned to their families. In many of these cases the perpetrator had taken an active, calculated role in creating a distorted story to foster alliances with the key adults who might offer the victim real protection.

In Kayla's case Daniel focused particularly on Kayla's mother, befriending her and promising to help Kayla become an Olympic-level athlete. Under the guise of doing what was "necessary" for her success, Daniel gained increasing unsupervised contact with, and control over, Kayla. Kayla's mother began to feel uncomfortable with the relationship but ended up deciding her worries were unjustified as Daniel worked hard to convince the key adults in Kayla's life that his actions made sense within the coach–athlete relationship.

> Trust your own intuition and observations: If you have persistent misgivings, don't allow the statements of the adult you are worried about dissuade you!

In other cases the perpetrator may lay the groundwork for discrediting the child, planting hints that she is untrustworthy and unreliable or "unruly and in need of discipline," casting doubt on any claims of abuse the child makes.

The statistics given in Chapter 2 show that the rate of disclosure by children, even once they're adults, is low, but some children do disclose. What brings them to that point?

PUBERTY

While we may not know all the factors that help individual children reach their disclosure tipping point, we do know that as they reach puberty their feelings of guilt and shame often increase and they begin to understand more fully that the behaviors the perpetrator is asking of them are widely considered inappropriate. Studies in 2008 by Rosaleen McElvaney at Dublin City University and others suggest that, no matter when the abuse began, becoming a teenager may represent a "critical period" for disclosure. By adolescence, children have usually developed emotionally and cognitively to the point where they can evaluate relationships from a societal perspective. This evaluation in turn produces what psychologists call "cognitive dissonance"—the mental discomfort or stress that results when someone is trying to reconcile two contradictory ideas, such as that an abuser who says he loves the child is doing something to the child that society considers extremely harmful. What they might have felt only uneasy about when younger now crystallizes into a societal taboo. Ultimately this thought process motivates teens to end what they now can see more clearly as an abusive relationship.

This expanding adolescent awareness was certainly a factor in Kayla's reaching her tipping point. By the time Kayla was 14, conflict was mounting between her and her mother, created by the tension between Kayla's recognition and her mother's suspicions that the relationship with Daniel was not as it should be:

Undated (age 14)

My phone was ringing. I could hear the catchy tune drifting down the stairs to my ears. I lurched from my seat, bounded up the steps two at a time to my room, and reached it on the last ring.

"Hello," I said, just a little bit breathless.

"Hey, baby," his voice said into my ear, and a hush came over my body. He had that effect on me. He was able to calm me or frighten me on the drop of a hat. I felt my heart rate slow.

"Why didn't you answer when I called earlier?" I heard the warning sounds in his voice. The hint of aggravation was enough to make me watch my tongue.

"I had cross-country practice, remember, babe? I told you about it. I'm doing it to stay in shape." I hoped it was the right answer. The truth was I had been with John. At wrestling. Big no-no.

"Oh. Is that why you sound so out of breath?"

"I'm not out of breath, I'm excited you called me, baby." I stroked his ego one syllable at a time. I had learned the dance by now. I knew all the twists and turns of a lie.

"Hmmm." I heard him mumble something into the phone that I didn't quite catch.

"I'll be at judo soon. Will you be there?" Of course I already knew the answer.

"Yah, I might show up. Depends on what you're gonna do afterwards."

*I knew this was a trick question. Brian always gave me a ride home from judo. But I could tell Daniel was restless. It had been a long time since we had been alone together. **I knew what he wanted, and I didn't want to give it to him** . . .*

"Baby, you know my mom will completely fucking flip. She's such a bitch. I'll probably be grounded for a week if you bring me home."

"Whatever. I'll see you tonight." The disgust in his voice stung, but not enough for me to tell the truth. That I didn't want to see him. That every day my life was becoming more and more a lie. Not just to my family and friends anymore, but to me.

Kayla's recollection captures the period of time when a child's secrets become less thinly veiled, as both her internal conflict about the relationship with the perpetrator mounts and people in her environment—in this case Kayla's mother—sense that something, although they are often not sure what, is terribly wrong. It is at this juncture, at the first suspicion that a relationship a child is in may be improper in some fashion, that those around the child need to know the signs of an inappropriate adult–child relationship, described in Chapter 2. **At this time adults must not ignore their instincts, but instead consider how best to address their suspicions directly with the child.** But this advice applies not just to adults. There is evidence that a majority of children who do disclose do so first to a friend or peer, particularly during adolescence.

PEERS AS CONFIDANTS

The fact that children begin to form close bonds with peers around puberty may explain why they often confide in a friend instead of an adult. At this age children are beginning to strive for independence, and this drive often includes a shift from entrusting parents with confidences to entrusting their friends with them. As we'll describe, although Kayla didn't disclose her abuse until a few years after she reached puberty, when she finally did so it was in fact to a peer. (See the box on page 63 for more research findings on the people to whom children often disclose CSA.)

> Researchers report that 40–80% of CSA victims say *a friend their own age* was the first, and sometimes the only, person they told, which can mean that the abuse stays shielded from adult caretakers and authorities who could intervene effectively.

What we need to understand is not just *when* kids are likely to break their silence but, perhaps even more important, what *they say* are the reasons that they are finally able to speak up. Paula Schaeffer, a researcher at Yale, and her forensic team asked children in 2011 how they came to tell someone about sexual abuse and why children

TO WHOM DO CHILDREN USUALLY DISCLOSE?

- As noted earlier, 40–80% of abused children disclose to a peer.
- Many children, particularly if younger, disclose their abuse first to parents, particularly their mother, according to Lindsay Malloy and colleagues at Florida International University in in 2013.
- Not surprisingly, the disclosure to a parent is more likely when the perpetrator is not a member of the family and also when the child expects the parent to be sympathetic.
- While studies of the rate of disclosure to educators and other professionals are less consistent in their findings, Sedlak found in 2010 that educators make up roughly 50% of the professional reports of child abuse made to authorities.

waited to disclose their abuse. They found that children *chose to tell* as a result of:

1. Some increased internal distress, such as nightmares or panic attacks.
2. Someone on the outside specifically asking about it.
3. Direct evidence of abuse (someone witnesses the child being hurt, a pregnancy occurs, etc.).

Obviously, the appropriate response to direct evidence of abuse is to ask about it and to follow up from there, the subject of Chapter 4. But how do you know that a child is suffering internally?

INCREASED INTERNAL DISTRESS

For Kayla, rising conflict at home stemmed from growing concerns on her mother's part about how much time Kayla was spending with Daniel, as well as her mother's observation of Kayla's increasing social isolation and preoccupations with weight—all changes that deeply troubled Kayla's mother and stepfather. While correctly reading these warning signs that all was not right with Kayla, without adequate knowledge about the prevalence and patterns of child sexual abuse, Kayla's mother continued to believe her daughter's denials and assurances that there was no need to worry about the relationship with Daniel. Kayla, for her part, was experiencing spiraling internal distress over the secretiveness of her relationship and the dual realities she now habitually had to contend with. Her social isolation, conflict with her mother, and preoccupations with her weight were all outward signs of this internal distress:

July 22, 2005 (age 15)

Dear God,

Hi. It's me again. How are you? I'm okay. We just got to Atlanta for the Junior Olympics. I weigh like 60 kg. This is the heaviest I've ever weighed. My doctor said yesterday it's because I'm a stress eater and things are really bad right now.

I'm worried about my family life, but I need to be worrying about competing. My mind is going crazy. I feel like a clutter brain. Like right now I'm writing and I can't really concentrate on what I'm writing about.

Later that night . . .

Well, I'm back. I went swimming with all the judo guys. We had a pretty good time. I'm still feeling dazed . . . like I don't know what's going on.

God, please help me find happiness with myself. I'm starting to get nervous about the tournament. I hope I do well.

Lord, please help me do the best that I can do. Please have things go over smoothly with my mom while I'm here. I love her, but from this point on in my life I'm going to try and find myself and make myself happy for a change.

Things aren't going too well for me. I might as well admit that I've sunk into a depression.

What seems like a good thing happens and then it's over and I'm so sad all of a sudden and I feel so alone and helpless. I feel like that a lot lately actually.

I'm not happy with myself and now I understand I can't be happy with anyone else because misery loves company.

I know that when I lie I shouldn't, God; please forgive me. It's become a natural thing now. I'm slowly killing myself with a web of lies.

You know something else, God, I always felt so bad for those kids who ever thought of suicide and looked at it as the only way out, but every day I find myself thinking about it more and more. And then even if I want to talk to someone I can't because I'm reminded that I'm all alone.

If I tried to talk to my mom we end up in a fight and then she'd throw me in the psych house.

If I try to talk to Daniel I feel he is the only person nowadays who listens to anything I say but still we argue like a married couple. If I tried to tell him, things would be awkward and he wouldn't know how hard to push me at practice and he'd be afraid to break me mentally which I'm very close to anyway. So I can't tell him.

So if I can't talk to anyone, I'll write and pray to you to help make it better.

Lord, I know there are a lot of kids out there who have it way worse than me and I know there are a lot of kids out there who deserve it a lot more than me, but God I need your help pulling out of the sadness.

I don't want to be like this anymore. God, I'm sorry. I'm going to try not to lie anymore. Please God I feel so alone.

I don't think things are ever going to be the same. But I know something has to change because I can't go on like this. I'm so weary and I'm so tired. I love judo, and I can't imagine my life without it.

Please help me get control and help me reach my goals. I want to be somebody special. I want to know that I went as far as I can go with Daniel by my side and I want to be a loyal player.

I need him no matter . . . look how good he's made me and I'm only 15. Please God let everything turn out all right. I don't want to be sad anymore.

Love Always,
Kayla

Unfortunately for those who care for them, children who are being abused do not all exhibit the same outward signs of internal distress, making it more difficult to discern when abuse might be the underlying cause. But the declining mental focus, forgetfulness, change in demeanor at school, and unexplained sleep difficulties and exhaustion listed in Chapter 2 are some common signals that a child may also be suffering from other types of worrisome emotional distress without directly saying anything about it. We've also seen abused children show unexplained nervousness when asked questions about a person who turned out to be their abuser, or start to become obsessed with pleasing or alternatively avoiding an adult in their life, or become unable to converse with friends and family about activities involving that adult. When asked about these behavioral changes, children may evade the questions or insist nothing is wrong, but again, these are signals of increased distress that you might use as ways to nudge them toward a disclosure tipping point if in fact they are being hurt by someone. Remember, however, that parents' suspicions are not correct all of the time and you need to respect repeated denials and not become an interrogator; your goal is to let your child know that you are both interested in what they have to say and attentive to it. With this stance, plus some professional assistance when needed, you will have the best chance of hearing what is really going on in your child's life. Here's an example from one of us (Blaise Aguirre):

"I was referred to Samantha, a 16-year-old high school junior whose mother was concerned about her increasing school avoidance. The problems had started in the spring of her sophomore year after a breakup with her boyfriend of 8 months. She had become sullen and withdrawn, but then had found a listener in her volleyball coach, a woman 'who was more like a friend than a coach.'

"Toward the end of the school year, she struggled to get up in time to go to school and started to withdraw from her friends, but summer seemed to fix everything, to her mother's relief. On returning to school in the fall of junior year, Samantha soon started to struggle again with attendance and seemed exhausted during the day. She did not admit to having any symptoms of depression, and it was initially not clear what was making it difficult for her to attend school. I asked her if she had spoken to her coach, as she had seemed to have found her supportive. She seemed unsettled by the question: 'Why do you want to know?'

"'I'm just curious,' I answered, noting her reaction.

"I asked her how she had been sleeping and she admitted that falling asleep had been difficult because she was 'playing things over and over' in her mind. She said that she was having nightmares, but that she did not feel comfortable telling me what they were about and that she was worried what people at school were saying about her. She spoke openly about school and her friends, but when I approached the subject of her coach the second time, she again appeared suspicious of my questioning and her leg started shaking.

"A few sessions later, after she had missed most of the week with vague stomach concerns, I asked her if I could speak to the school counselor and the coach, and she started to cry. I asked her if something had happened between her and the coach, and she put her head in her lap and sobbed uncontrollably.

"I brought her mother into the session to share my worry that, although I did not have direct information, the nightmares, school avoidance, and her reactions to mentions of the coach warranted further investigation. In the context of a reassuring and supportive family response, Samantha admitted that the coach had been helpful at first, but that then her behavior started to confuse her as it became more physical in an unwanted way, but that she had not known where to turn.

"Her opening up initially brought with it shame, guilt, and anger. We developed a treatment plan that involved dealing directly with what had happened. This, together with the school's suspension of the coach and pending investigation, led to a marked reduction in symptoms and a gradual return to a happier and engaged self."

In cases like Samantha's, adults often assume they're dealing with normal teenage angst. Samantha had, after all, gone through a painful breakup, so it would have been understandable that she had difficulty facing her ex and her friends every day at school. How do parents know when they're dealing with symptoms of adolescent development and when these symptoms indicate something else?

Signs of Abuse or "Normal" Childhood Angst?

It's perfectly understandable, and common, to ask yourself whether emotional and behavioral changes in your child indicate a problem or are just part of a normal developmental phase. For many youth, the teenage years in particular are synonymous with drama. Although children of all ages face challenges, teens in particular must address new experiences that involve relationships with their peers, like having difficulties with girlfriends or boyfriends; daily decisions about what to wear to create the "right" image; which friendships to pursue; and how to handle doing poorly on a test or on the soccer field.

A massive surge in hormones complicates everything, making teens more sensitive at a time when they are particularly self-conscious and lack the skill set to manage the events that arise.

Episodes of sadness, irritability, anxiety, frustration, and feeling overwhelmed are not unusual but shouldn't last long if they are just part of typical development. Here are a few red flags to watch for:

- Emotional distress that lasts longer than a few hours or a few days.
- A sudden change from the behavior that's typical for the teen's peer group.
- A sudden change in the teen's own typical behavior.

Although none of the specific behaviors listed below are in and of themselves symptoms of a psychological disorder, they are concerning and warrant closer attention if they persist for your child:

- A significant decrease in enjoyment and time spent with friends and family.
- A significant decrease in school performance or school attendance.
- Sudden and sustained problems with memory, attention, or concentration.
- Sudden and significant changes in sleeping patterns.
- Persistent physical symptoms, such as stomachaches and headaches.
- Moodiness, with frequent crying and irritability lasting for weeks.
- Frequent, uncharacteristic verbal or physical fights, enduring oppositional behavior, or disobedience.
- Substance use, particularly in isolation.
- Sudden changes in eating behavior.
- Increasing isolation and withdrawal from friends and activities and interacting with others only on social media.

The bottom line: If you see signs of emotional distress in your child, you must ask the child about it. But how?

STEPS TO TAKE
WHEN YOU SUSPECT CHILD SEXUAL ABUSE

What Kayla's parents did not and could not have known, because of insufficient public awareness at the time, was that Kayla's emotional and behavioral difficulties were in fact the symptoms of her involvement in an abusive relationship with Daniel. They also didn't know at the time that there are some *dos* and *don'ts* for how to approach a child with concerns about abuse, particularly when the suspected adult is a trusted and important figure in the child's life. Not appreciating the central role that Daniel played in Kayla's life, and still assuming that Kayla would tell them "the truth" if something inappropriate was going on, Kayla's parents continued to trust that their daughter was suffering from the predictable stresses of adolescence. Kayla's mom later recounted both her suspicions of abuse and the way in which Daniel actively worked to keep her fears at bay:

"I really *thought* I knew Daniel; after all he was the sensei at Renshuden Club, a prestigious judo school not far from our home in Middletown, Ohio. He was charming, entertaining all of us with his silly jokes and imitations, and also coached alongside his father, who was a gentle guy with an Irish lilt. All of this made him seem safe . . . trustworthy . . .

"Over time Daniel spent more and more time with us as a family; he rode in our car to competitions in distant cities and shared meals and did everything with us that we did as a family. He vacationed with us because judo tournaments doubled as our holidays. He babysat all of my kids and sometimes gave Kayla a lift to practice. Over one summer he even built a retaining wall and a pool in our backyard.

"Truthfully, it did bother me when he snapped at practice, kicked Kayla in the back of the legs, and spoke to her as if she were a dog . . . but he did that to other kids, and besides, I thought to myself 'wasn't that what coaches did?' It also unnerved me when he began carping at Kayla about her diet, her clothing, her hair, her friends, but by then people were talking about her as a future Olympian, and I thought that maybe those two things went together—his demanding control and her perfectionism— and that this combination was the only one possible to make an Olympic champion . . ."

There's that distorted story line again. Kayla's mom and stepdad were no match for a perpetrator who had skillfully worked his way into a trusted position and a place of great importance in Kayla's life and that of her entire family. Looking back, Kayla agreed:

Daniel was one of my mum's friends, he babysat me and my brother and sister, he came over for family barbecues . . . he coached me to two national titles before my 15th birthday, and later I realized that he had used our coach–athlete relationship to abuse the trust of both me and my entire family.

So what do we know about the optimal conditions for disclosure? We know that the following conditions make it significantly more likely that children will disclose abuse:

- Being asked directly about experiences of abuse, sometimes more than once.
- Knowing that they are likely to be believed and not blamed.
- Believing they will be protected by the adult they disclose to.
- Believing they will be able to maintain a sense of control over the process of disclosure, in terms of both preserving their anonymity (not being identified until they are ready) and maintaining confidentiality (controlling who knows). At times this need for control extends to worrying about what will happen to the person who has been hurting them. This critical sense of control is discussed in detail in Chapter 4.

Be Direct and Gently Persistent

We've seen over and over in practice what researchers have found as well: Directly asking children if they have been sexually abused, in a supportive yet persistent manner, increases the chances of disclosure. In fact, showing an interest in the key relationships in their lives itself increases the likelihood that they will tell you if one of these relationships becomes abusive. Children we've seen after disclosure often say the same thing: They finally told someone after being prompted rather than because they independently and spontaneously chose to do so. It's also important to bear in mind, however, that many youth initially deny that they've been sexually abused, even with repeated questioning, and then respond truthfully only at a later date, when their heightened personal distress and desperation to end the abuse lead to breaking their silence. This was the case with Kayla. So if your nagging doubts don't disappear after your first inquiry, and especially if your child continues to exhibit signs of distress and poor functioning, continue to let the child know that you're worried about her and that your worries include whether her relationship with "X" has become a problem.

It's understandable to find the idea of your child being sexually abused so horrifying that your first reaction to a suspicion may be to second-guess what you sense or see or to deny it altogether. We can't stress strongly enough how necessary it is not to yield to that temptation. We're also not suggesting that you start seeing evil around every corner. But when you have a strong negative feeling about a person who has become far too entwined in your child's life, or you're seeing any of the signs of emotional distress we've listed so far, pay attention. Maybe parents' hope that they'll get a negative answer to queries about whether someone is harming their child, along with the general belief that we as parents would know immediately if our child was being hurt, is why many adults beat around the bush, initially asking questions that are so ambiguous or open ended that the child can easily say nothing is wrong. Other parents signal to the child, no matter how subtly, that they want to hear that nothing is wrong, and that's what the child tells them. Additionally, the fact that the relationship in question often involves an already known and trusted adult can make it feel inappropriate to a parent to even be asking about possible improprieties.

We've seen many parents misinterpret their child's apparent attachment to a person who was later revealed to have abused him. For example, when a child and an adult become involved in a relationship that starts to take up an inordinate amount of the child's focus, time,

> When evidence of a problem is before you, do whatever you can to resist the temptation to second-guess and dismiss your suspicion.

and emotional energy, parents can innocently but mistakenly jump to the conclusion that it's the child pursuing additional contact with an admired teacher, coach, or neighbor. When the perpetrator of sexual abuse is someone well known to you and a person of importance to your child but also someone respected by the larger community, it can be particularly difficult to persist in your suspicions absent any clear corroborating evidence or information. But again, it's critical to follow your instincts that there may be more going on than is being acknowledged. Sometimes you need to read between the lines of what children say or pay attention to what they do, instead of just what they say. For example, we commonly hear this type of statement from children who come to see us at McLean following the disclosure of abuse:

> "My mom definitely knew something was up, but all she said to me was to stop talking so much about X and accused me of having a crush on him and all of that . . . boy, did she have that wrong. I was really hoping she would confront him or just forbid me to see him again, but I also realized she couldn't do that . . . he was so close to all my friends and everyone else in my family."

In a case like this, the victim's mother obviously noticed something awry in how her daughter was behaving toward the abuser. While it's understandable to be uncomfortable to the point of rejecting the thoughts that come to mind about the possibility of abuse, we strongly encourage you to step back and muster your courage; resist the temptation to avoid or shrug off your concerns and ask your child gently and persistently whether this person is harming her in any way.

When confronting a child about your suspicions that he or she is being sexually abused,

Instead of saying . . .	Say . . .
"Is something going on with you and X?" (implies consent)	"Is X hurting you in any way?"
"Did I see you and X touching?" (implies consent)	"I know X is important to you, and I'm also worried about how I see him acting toward you."
"Why is X always calling you? I have a good mind to report X to the school and let them investigate." (threatening loss of control)	"Lots of times what starts out as a healthy relationship can go in a harmful direction. I'm worried that is happening with you and X."
"I think you've become too involved with X." (judgmental of child)	"I'm concerned that X is putting too much pressure on you as his star athlete/student."

It took a confluence of several factors for Kayla to reach the tipping point of disclosing: (1) a greater awareness over time of the impropriety of the relationship with Daniel, (2) hearing from team-mates that Daniel was in a romantic relationship that he was hiding, (3) increased despair of finding a way to change her relationship to Daniel without losing this critical relationship altogether, and (4) anguish over the double existence she was leading. These factors in combination helped Kayla realize that staying silent might no longer be an option:

> When you live a lie, when you lie to the people who are closest to you day in and day out, it eats away at you. I was at the point where I was ready to run away, I was ready to kill myself, or I was going to have to say something . . .

It is at this tipping point, when children are close to disclosure, that being asked about whether an abusive relationship exists is most likely to lead to a revelation. But it can be very difficult to know when this point has been reached. Kayla's mother hopes that her memory of what Kayla was like right before she disclosed will help other parents recognize the signs:

> "I remember you were superemotional. You stopped having contact with Daniel. You seemed very depressed and quiet. You were so quiet.
>
> "When we talked to Jimmy about you going there [months before Kayla's disclosure], you would bounce between depressed and crying to excited and hopeful. You seemed happy. It was almost as if you had a plan and a way out. But then you would dissolve into tears and seem lifeless.
>
> "I definitely didn't think you were about to tell me what you told me. I just felt it was a hard time for you because you were ready to move on but scared about the process."

The challenge of knowing how, what, and when to ask in these circumstances, however, is obviously no small matter and therefore should be considered by parents and caretakers before they come face-to-face with these problems in the course of daily life. The examples given earlier show the often subtle differences between language that might elicit a disclosure and language that can feel blaming or threatening to the child. Another important factor is to be as specific as you can in crafting your questions and describing your observations. If you initially meet with a denial from your child, you might follow up with questions like these:

> "Honey, I keep feeling like something is really wrong in your relationship with X. Do you think you could talk to me about this?"

> "You're still talking a lot about X . . . Are you upset about something that he is doing or saying?"

> "This is the fourth time this week you've gone in early to review your math homework with Mr. X . . . This really concerns me, and I worry that he's putting too much pressure on you to excel."

Effective prompts and questions don't necessarily need to be about sexual abuse per se but can be generally about the young person's psychological distress and well-being. Rosaleen McElvaney found in her studies that the questioning itself acts as an external force, often adding the pressure the child or teen needs to finally divulge her secret. So don't be afraid to persist!

Communicate Your Support

As the suggestions of what to say to your child to elicit a disclosure show, expressing that you're there to support and help your child may be all that is needed to create a tipping point. But social support in general also increases disclosure, especially during adolescence. A child who has a trusted group of friends, teammates, classmates, or extended family may feel more willing and able to divulge abuse because he feels like he's not alone, he'll likely be believed, and his experiences with those around him include being helped when needed.

Increasing the level of informal supervision of your child is another way to create the tipping point. Suggesting, for example, that a friend or grandparent instead of a coach or teacher handle the carpool puts your child in proximity to an adult who may inspire a confidence, or at least make the child feel less alone. Those who sexually abuse children often target youth who seem isolated, and having to keep the abuse a secret makes children feel even more alone. The saying that there is safety in numbers is true in more ways than one. Could a friend accompany your child to an early practice or homework hour? Being with a peer may, again, stimulate a disclosure, but at the very least the child will not be alone and unprotected.

In all conversations with your child intended to uncover abuse, it's essential to communicate that you know that sometimes kids don't speak up for fear that no one will believe them and that you would never want that fear to prevent your child from talking to you. It's important to note here as well that,

> If you suspect your child is being abused, anything you can do to increase his or her overall social support or informal supervision may help create a tipping point.

while false disclosures of child sexual abuse are relatively rare, they do occur, and all you can do is make sure that you respond to whatever you hear nonjudgmentally and with an open mind; most of the time what you hear will be true even though at times it may be very hard to accept.

It's estimated that somewhere between 4 and 8% of allegations of child sexual abuse (under 10% across studies according to *Darkness to Light* in 2017) are untrue, with a majority of these claims involving custody disputes in which allegations are first made by the adults involved. It can then be difficult for the child to discriminate between what is false and what is true, especially if the allegations involve events that took place when the child was very young.

It's important to realize that a child who is being abused is on high alert at all times. Her psychological defense system may be primed to protect her secret because staying silent is tightly woven into her strategy for protecting herself—even though it, paradoxically, allows the abuse to continue. So, when you're trying to draw out the truth about a relationship that the child is involved in, you may have to navigate a fine line between being specific and

> Be sure your child knows that when you ask about sexual abuse, you're truly interested in hearing what she has to say, even if it involves someone you know and feel close to.

being open. This is why we suggested on page 72 that you follow a statement like "You've been talking a lot about X" with "Is something bothering you about him?" Asking just "Why are you talking so much about X?" may elicit a defensive response of "I'm NOT talking about him so much." And suggesting or insisting that you know "the truth" before you are told not only runs the risk of pushing the child further into a self-protective silence but also does not leave room for the possibility that you may be wrong in your suspicions. Remember, the goal is always to let your child know that your concerns are based on what you've observed or been told by others who know the child well and that you're looking to your child to help you understand whether an adult is hurting her.

Always bear in mind that young children especially can be suggestible. It's important not to become suspicious in a way that makes your child worry when there is in fact no danger. You need to strike a balance, communicating neither that all adults can be trusted nor that no adults can be trusted—and that you are open to talking with your child about her reactions to all of the adults in her life.

Communicate Your Protectiveness

One of the most common concerns of children on the brink of disclosure is whether they will be protected by whomever they disclose to. In instances where the perpetrator has directly threatened their safety, or that of other family members, protecting your child may necessitate talking to law enforcement and obtaining protective services, often in the form of a restraining order. But often the perpetrator's threats are more subtle and imply there will be retribution in the form of a withdrawal of privileges and support, such as coaching, the chance to be an altar boy, or tutoring services. Adults need to anticipate this possibility and, as part of the conversation, let the child know they'll make sure she doesn't "lose out" on anything following the disclosure. Specifically, this means telling the child that they will help her find a safer replacement to provide what she is currently getting from the perpetrator; in Kayla's case this took the form of finding new coaches in Boston so that her athletic goals were not dashed. In Chapter 4 we talk more about understanding how important it is to child victims that they retain control of the situation, including not losing the perceived benefits of the relationship with their abuser.

Help Them Anticipate the Fallout

In Chapter 4 we also review in detail what are the likely outcomes, in terms of legally prosecuting the perpetrator and enlisting the help of child protective services, when a child of a specific age discloses sexual abuse. It's not always possible for a child to have her revelations kept confidential, either because the person she tells is mandated to report the allegations or because the person she tells decides it is not in the child's best interest to keep the abuse undisclosed. Whatever the realities may be, part of talking effectively with a child you suspect may be at the tipping point for disclosure is to be direct in your assurances that you know these issues exist and you will look into them carefully. However, don't promise that "nothing will happen," as that is typically not accurate. Rather, let the child you are talking to or working with be part of the process of finding out the rules in your state and remind her that you are "in this together."

IF YOU SEE SOMETHING, SPEAK UP

By "see something," we obviously don't mean just directly witnessing abuse or its consequences (such as pregnancy). We mean observing that something is wrong. It's essential for parents, caregivers, and peers to follow the guideline *"if you see something that looks or feels wrong to you between an adult and a child . . . speak up."* Awareness education programs that target preteens and adolescents, as well as adults, are shaping up to be powerful and necessary prevention tools in encouraging earlier disclosures. The status and availability of existing prevention and awareness programs for CSA are discussed in Chapter 8.

For Kayla, while she privately wrote about the wish to be discovered, her relationship with Daniel and with judo made losing him impossible to contemplate as well. This intricate balance drove Kayla to experience mood swings and more frequent suicidal thinking and to display erratic behaviors, some of which were visible to the outside world if only those around her had understood the possible significance of what they were seeing. For example, Kayla recalls a time when she reacted in the extreme to her parents' refusal to let her go to Daniel's house one weekend:

[age 13–14]

There was even a point in time where my mom . . . I didn't clean my room or something, and my mom said I couldn't go to the team get-together Daniel was having that weekend. I lost it, I went off, and my dad had to hold me down. He had to restrain me. And

I called the cops on them and I told them, "My dad, he fucking, he held me down," and the cops put me in my place, but in my mind I couldn't believe that they wouldn't let me go, and I was frantic, I was panicked. I literally had a meltdown because they wouldn't let me go to his house that weekend.

It happened during a time of adolescence, and I think that's why it was confusing for my parents because when I was 8 years old, 10 years old, I was this great bubbly personality. I was a pleaser. And then almost the same time I hit puberty, I started to get a little more angsty and a little more like "Well, I'm not gonna listen to you . . .

Do you ever feel completely out of control, like you just don't have your hands on the wheel? That's exactly how I felt, like I had no control over my life. I was so beyond infuriated that I didn't have the control to do what I wanted to do and especially because I knew he was going to be pissed. I'm sure he was furious with me and super disappointed . . . and then he would turn it and say, "Well, your mom's such a fucking bitch." He would say I was terrible, I was not a good person because I didn't clean my room, and then that my mom was not a good person for using that against me.

Kayla's mother recalls being completely at a loss to explain her daughter's extreme reaction to being told she couldn't go to Daniel's house:

> "I don't remember what it was about at all, probably about, you know, cleaning your room or something like that. I just know that I told you that you couldn't go to Daniel's and you became very upset over that. I know that it was because he would become angry with you. And, you know, we being your parents, we said that we really didn't care if he became angry with you because we were the ones that were governing your life, not him."

Unfortunately, at that time there were still not enough red flags to move Kayla's mother to action:

> "I just thought, what the hell is going on? I just didn't know what to think. I just was like, what is going on with her? I just . . . I didn't know what to think."

A year or so later, Kayla's parents were seeing some pretty startling behavior from her—and definitely a shift from her old "bubbly" self, and yet they didn't know what was operating under the surface, as exemplified by the following excerpt from her journals from the year before Kayla disclosed:

July 23, 2005 (age 15)

Dear God,

Hi. How are you? I'm doing better today. Well, actually today was a lot worse. I fought with my mom and Daniel, and they both said some things that made me feel like crap.

I was crying at the tournament because my mom and Daniel got really pissed off. He told me I might as well quit judo. It hurts my feelings, and all day today I've been trying to talk to him, but he won't talk to me. I'm angry and frustrated.

Today when things got really bad again I thought about killing myself. I thought about how everyone would feel if I did something like that. I don't know if Daniel would even give a damn. It hurts to think about things like that. Sometimes he's so immature he's like my age. I don't understand. I think I need to just let go.

Tomorrow I fight. Please let me do good, God.

I'm so angry, God. And I'm so sad. I don't know why. Life just doesn't get any easier. I have to fight tooth and nail with everyone to play judo and I'm beginning to wonder if it's ever going to be worth it. I don't know.

I feel so alone and depressed right now. My life is like an endless cycle of anger and sadness. Lately I feel no triumph or happiness. I see only the negative, and I can't stand to look at myself in the mirror.

*I hate myself. I hate who I've become. Please God help me. I don't want to feel like this anymore. Please help make things better. **Please let someone notice what is going on and make it stop.***

Love Always,
Kayla

It's important to note that Kayla realizes her parents were probably confused by the change in her and believes it was possible that they didn't understand the significance of the change because it had taken place over a long period of time. What if they had said something when they first saw the signs of such drastic changes in their child's demeanor?

Parents and others rightfully ask how they can be sure they *are* seeing something. As with other facets of disclosing or discovering sexual abuse, it's often difficult (if not impossible) to be certain. But there are two yardsticks by which we can get an idea of whether a child is likely to be suffering sexual abuse: (1) behavior that is known clinically to be associated with such abuse and (2) a knowledge of the individual child.

Behaviors That Often Indicate Child Sexual Abuse

So far in this book we've listed the signs of increasing internal distress that can be associated with trauma in order to help you determine whether your child may be suffering from undisclosed sexual abuse. The more you know about the signs and circumstances that can be red flags, the more likely that you can help your child reach the tipping point, if in fact she is harboring a secret of this kind. Childhood victims, who are trying to survive as best they can in a circumstance that feels both confusing and hopeless, ultimately rely on others noticing and asking questions in order to make a full disclosure as soon as possible after the abuse begins. So here is another group of indications— common, but not necessarily all-inclusive or definitive, behaviors that can be associated with experiencing sexual abuse:

- A preoccupation with a specific adult to the exclusion of peers and family.
- Avoidance of formerly enjoyed activities or activities involving a particular adult.
- An increase in aggressive behaviors toward parents and/or siblings in response to efforts to limit a specific adult relationship.
- An increase in defiance of age-appropriate rules and limits, particularly as regards a specific adult.
- The child's acting and behaving older than his or her chronological age.
- An increase in developmentally inappropriate sexualized behaviors and activities.
- The seeking of support from peers concerning related issues, as in statements like "I have a friend who has a problem with . . ."

All of these signs call for gentle, persistent questioning about whether the child is being touched or treated inappropriately in any way that we've described.

> Don't use knowledge of symptoms that can be associated with child sexual abuse to make your own diagnosis. Instead, use observing these symptoms as a reason to ask your child about them judiciously and without accusations. The goal is to open a dialogue that will elicit the child's disclosure of any abuse that is occurring.

The Importance of Knowing the Child

To have a good sense for whether a suspicion of child sexual abuse may be accurate, it's also important to know the child. Often it is only the people in a child's everyday life who bear witness to the quality of the child's relationship with a particular adult and thus have the first-hand information necessary to raise and support a suspicion. As a parent you have the opportunity to notice if your child is acting unusual around a specific coach or teacher and to then ask relevant questions and also gather impressions about that person and his or her conduct from other people in your community network.

In contrast, speculations that abuse is the root cause of a child's emotional difficulties can't be considered particularly reliable—and may even be ill advised. When CSA was first recognized as a prevalent problem, we learned a hard lesson that children, especially very young children, can indeed be influenced by adults who repeatedly suggest that they may have been abused by someone in their past, particularly when they are at an age when memory can be unreliable.

Without direct knowledge of the individual child, a physician or other health care provider observing emotional difficulties could mistakenly ascribe them to nonexistent sexual abuse or, more important, disregard the possibility when sexual abuse is actually occurring, as illustrated in a medical note from Kayla's records after she spent the summer traveling internationally for judo competitions with relatively little adult supervision or support. Knowing nothing specific about Daniel, her family doctor, upon examining Kayla, attributes all of her emotional symptoms to the stress of being a high-level, competitive judoka even though

> What we are aiming for is to neither shy away from our suspicions when these are based on observation nor create suspicions out of whole cloth.

THE RISK OF ASKING PROBING QUESTIONS WITHOUT CORROBORATING EVIDENCE

In the early 1990s, along with an increasing awareness that CSA was widespread and often went unreported, therapists began asking probing questions that suggested a client might have been victimized without any direct information about a troubling relationship or other indicators that the child had been harmed. At that time a flood of self-help books along with the rise of "recovered memory therapy" led to a number of well-publicized, false allegations of CSA that were later recanted. In her pioneering work at that time, Elizabeth Loftus demonstrated that in approximately 25% of her subjects, false memories could be *implanted* via discussion and suggestion so that an individual later "recalls" an event that he believes happened that, in fact, had not. There are also some corroborating accounts and scientific evidence that the mind is capable of repressing traumatic memories.

Due to these uncertainties, there is a consensus in the field that therapists should never suggest to a child that something "must have happened" to him or her, especially in the absence of any disclosure or other possible corroborating evidence of sexual abuse, which can include information such as the fact that the child's siblings were abused by X or that a teacher in the school the child attends has been discovered to have hurt other pupils of the same age. And even in this latter instance, one would inquire but never suggest or insist that this particular child has been victimized. Asking about whether something is going on, or if a child has been hurt by a known perpetrator, is different from insisting that something "must have happened" before a child may be ready to talk and has possibly not suffered CSA.

she has already been prescribed Prozac for depression, noted in an earlier physical:

9.13.2005 Doctor's Visit

Patient is 15 years old. Comes in today for follow-up on fatigue and depression. Recently, starting on Prozac weekly because of increasing depression that was first marked on her sports physical on July 21, 2005. We started Prozac weekly, which she has tolerated well. She feels that it is helping but she is still feeling stressed and overwhelmed. She's a world-class judo athlete and travels a lot. She also has recently started running cross-country. She states that last night she had judo practice, cross country practice, and four hours of homework and felt a bit overwhelmed. She does have a history of hypoglycemia in the past, and she has not been eating a snack after school prior to practice either for cross-country or judo. I've asked to look at her hypoglycemic diet and try to get back on track here. She may be having low sugar reactions, which are probably complicating the stress and anxiety.

Without any contextual information from those who knew Kayla well, this doctor had no idea that her visible emotional distress might be related to ongoing abuse and did not ask any specific screening questions about relationship violence or violations. While Kayla's case is somewhat atypical in that she traveled a great deal without her parents and saw many different physicians and specialists, in general parents should share any ongoing concerns they have with their child's doctor and maintain continuity as much as possible with a physician who knows the child, has a relationship with the family, and is provided up-to-date information about recent changes and concerns.

IF YOU HEAR SOMETHING, RESPOND

Children often make tentative disclosures before making unambiguous revelations of abuse. As noted above, they might say they have a friend who is having a problem to feel out how you would likely react if they disclosed their own abuse. Or they might tell an adult smaller, less worrisome details first or give the adult a newspaper or magazine story to read that suggests they are scared or being hurt in some fashion. This is an opportunity to nudge your child to the tipping point of disclosure. Do your best not to ignore or toss off any overture about anything resembling possible sexual abuse. If you react calmly, with concern but not alarm, your child will hopefully sense that you're open to hearing more. We suggest that you invite your child to say more by asking for details and expressing the desire to be supportive and protective. If you realize later that you may have missed such an opportunity, go back to your child, apologize for being distracted, and ask what he wanted to talk about.

REACHING THE TIPPING POINT

The triggers to disclosure can be as simple as a friend in the child's environment asking her timely questions or as complicated as the child running into a physical or emotional complication that she can no longer handle in secrecy, such as an unplanned pregnancy. In Kayla's case, turning 16 brought her troubles even further into the forefront of consciousness, and she marked that milestone with a particularly haunting entry in her beloved journal:

My 16th Birthday

Wolf in a Blanket

I open my eyes and look at the clock. 2:08 A.M. is flashing in bright blue on the nightstand. The house is quiet. So quiet. Happy Birthday, Kayla, I think. 16. Hmmm. Only 2 years till you're an adult. Hard to believe considering you may as well be 35.

I slip out of bed and head to the bathroom. In the hallway I listen to hear everyone's breath. Lisa, Sara, and Jasmine are just across the hall. Doing judo twice a day has exhausted them. I hear Sara's chainsaw snore and know they are out.

In the bathroom I look in the mirror. You don't look any older. But maybe that's a good thing. He did say he liked you more when you were thinner and younger. I grab the soft flesh around my abdomen and bite my lip. Growing up is hard. I can do better. I can make him love me more. I swig some mouthwash and pinch my cheeks even though it will be dark. I am not allowed to wear makeup, but I've seen Lisa do it and he looks at her . . . bitch.

*I tiptoe to his bedroom. His door is slightly open. **A sign for me and only me.** I can hear the hum of the AC going full blast. His room is the only room with one. The rest of the house is full of sticky children under thin sheets and buzzing fans. The hall light is on, and I don't want that to be what wakes him, so I slide in as fast and silent as I can. He is a giant snoring mound under the covers. The wolf blanket is covering his belly while his barrel chest and bald head gleam in the hallway light. I close the door all the way.*

When I slide into bed next to him he reaches for me and I fit right into his arms as he fits right into my cold, dead heart. This is where I shut down. This is where I go to my place. He is rubbing my back and I am leaving this world.

The wolf blanket was always my favorite blanket. I always looked into the wolf's eyes and knew he was a loner. I could hear his ghostly howl from right there in the bedroom. He was howling for me. For my soul. For my pain. I am saying my prayers.

> Now I lay me down to sleep
> I pray the Lord my soul to keep
> if I should die before I wake
> I pray the Lord my Soul to take.

Please God take my soul. Take it out of this body and put it with you. Put it with the devil.

Put it anywhere but here with this man.

"I love you." I say.

"I love you too, babe," he whispers.

"Can I stay with you tonight? Please."

"You know you can't. No one can know our secret, Kayla. Come on, you're old enough to know this by now."

"I know, I just love you so much. I want to sleep with you. All night. Just once. I want to wake up with you."

"You will. Someday soon, baby bird. Now go to bed."

I lie in bed and can't sleep. I am dirty. I need a shower. I am sticky. My mouth is dry. I am restless. Tomorrow I will go home and kiss my mom. We will have a pool party for my 16th birthday. I will blow out the candles and smile. Everyone will drink and laugh and be merry. I will drink too. And my cold dead heart will beat on inside.

Kayla's confusion and torment continued as she tried to figure out how to flee her private prison of shame and secrecy. After finding out from peers that Daniel had been lying to her and was romantically involved with a woman his own age, Kayla steeled herself to try to break up with him in a way that would not call further attention to their relationship. She tried valiantly to end their sexual relationship and, as reflected in her journal entries, found it nearly impossible to end things on her own:

April 3, 2007 (age 16)

Dear God,

Nice storm. Well I finally ended things. I'm not sure how I feel. I mean I feel better with myself, but sometimes I just get so sad and I remember all the good times. I mean I remember the bad times too, but for some reason they just make me sadder.

God, please let me be okay. If I stay here and he doesn't let me go, I'm afraid. I'm afraid of who I'll become. I can't go back. Let the storm end.

Love Always,
Kayla

Later that day . . .

Dear God,

I know I just wrote you, but I feel so restless and sad. I want to call him because he's the only one I can talk to, but I know I can't. And Brian won't understand. I just feel so alone, God, and it leads me to second-guess myself. I can't live with him, and I can't live without him. I think I need him but then I think "Fuck him." Please help me, God. Let me be strong and give me the courage to change my life.

Love Always,
Kayla

*   *   *

The last month has felt like a year. Going to judo every night feels like ripping out my soul. The only good thing is to see Daniel hurting as much as me. He looks like he hasn't slept in a month. He has started binge drinking again. Some days he shows up to my morning workouts with Brian and just stares pleadingly at me. I ignore him. I ignore his calls. His texts. I delete his voice mails without listening. Every night I lay my head down to sleep and I can't. The panic and hysteria set it. The tears come. But I don't break. I don't call him.

Everyone is beginning to notice my complete and utter hate for Daniel. They look on but never say anything. When Brian asks,

I just say we're in a fight. I don't say about what or why. I keep my answers short and my heart walled off. If I feel something, anything, I know I will break and that my chance will be gone forever. I hold on tight to his betrayal. I wear it like a cloak. I let myself feel that hurt and it fuels my resolve.

We have to go to Puerto Rico for a tournament. I don't want to travel with Daniel, but I don't want to raise alarms. I am still trying to figure out my plan.

Puerto Rico, April 2007 (age 16)

As soon as I step off the plane the heat hits me hard. It's sweltering. Daniel has been drinking the entire flight down. He brought a bottle of Jack Daniels from customs on the plane and it is almost empty by the time we arrive. He reeks of panic.

Diana, Jess, and Brian are worried. We will be meeting up with the rest of team USA tomorrow, and they know that Daniel can't be seen like this. He is a mess. He threw up on himself in the cab ride to the hotel. The airport lost his bags. They decide we have to send him home. While we check in to the hotel, Jess and Diana go to the airport to try and change his ticket, and Brian goes to the local mall to buy Daniel a change of clothes. Daniel and I are alone for the first time in months.

"Baby bird, please talk to me. I'm so sorry, Kayla. I love you so fucking much. I can't live without you." He slurs.

I look at him. For the first time in my life I am in control of this relationship. I think I love him and when I see him like this I crack.

"Okay, Daniel. It's going to be okay. Jess and Diana are going to send you home. You have to get help. If you get help, we can talk, okay? But I can't watch you like this. I can't do it. You have to take care of yourself, and then we can talk, okay?" I say.

"Okay, baby bird. Anything you want. I'll do anything you fucking want. Don't leave me. I need you. I need you so fucking much."

I start to cry. "I need you too, Daniel. But I need you to be strong. I need you to get better, and then it will be okay. Everything will be okay." I lie. It kills me. Nothing is okay.

"Okay, baby bird, okay. Come lay down with me . . . just for a little bit."

I lie with him on the bed in Puerto Rico. It will be the last time he ever touches me.

In the end it was one of Kayla's teammates, a teammate who she was close to and who gave her rides home after practice, that succeeded in pushing through her silence by persisting with the questions that needed to be asked. Ultimately it took both Kayla, who was ready and desperate to flee her abuse, and a concerned friend who cared enough not to be daunted in his pursuit of the truth:

> And in just this way the secrecy and shame that surrounded my 4 years of sexual abuse, abuse I had kept secret from everyone, came to an end.
>
> By that time I hated what Daniel was doing to me but had not been able to think of a way out, alternately loving and hating this person who had become the center of my success and happiness.
>
> In school, I kept trying to just "be normal," but my double life took its toll; and by the end, I had pulled away from friends, demolished my relationship with my mother and stepfather, and was toying with thoughts of suicide.
>
> Although I was already a rising star in judo, I began hating the sport that was so tangled up with Daniel. I had won championships by this time and yet thought every single day about quitting.
>
> And then Brian finally realized that something was terribly wrong and this time decided to not once again let me ride home silently staring out the window and in tears.

Kayla recollects these painful moments in detail, when she finally broke through the prison of silence, shame, and fear she had lived in since the age of 12:

> Brian and I are in the car. We are on the long drive home from nationals in Florida. I have eaten so much I've been sick. I keep eating even though it doesn't fill me. Nothing does.
>
> It's raining. Brian is asking me questions about Daniel and he won't stop.
>
> "What happened, Kayla?" he asks.
>
> "He just makes me uncomfortable."
>
> "What happened?"
>
> "I just can't train with him anymore. He's made a move on me, and I can't take it."
>
> "What happened?"
>
> Silence.

"What happened? Tell me. What happened?"

"He's been fucking me since I was 12, okay?" I scream. "Is that what you want? There it is. He's been fucking me since I was 12."

He hits the windshield and it shatters. Just like my life.

*   *   *

We pull over to a rest stop and Brian makes me call my mom. He makes me leave a voice message because she is flying home. I repeat it. "Daniel has been having sex with me for years." I am numb.

*   *   *

My phone is ringing. I tell Brian I have to use the bathroom. In the stall I answer.

"Hello."

"What the fuck have you done, Kayla?" Daniel says. He doesn't sound angry. Just quiet and subdued.

"Daniel, I'm so sorry. I don't know why I said anything. I'll take it back. I'm so so sorry." I sob.

"One of us isn't going to make it out of this alive, Kayla," he says.

"I love you," I say. He hangs up.

I don't remember the rest of the ride.

When she hears her daughter's message and the reality and extent of the abuse at last become undeniable, Kayla's mother smashes in Daniel's car windows and goes straight to the police. Daniel is arrested before Kayla even has a moment to take in what is happening. She recalls from this time feeling both guilty and unsure about whether the abuse was really all her fault and whether she still loved the man who had been her mentor and constant companion for so many years.

Then within a matter of weeks, Kayla's mother made a stunning move: sending her daughter off to Boston to create distance from the publicity in Ohio and allow Kayla to continue her training with the Pedros, a father and son team with significant stature in the judo community. And as so often happens when the secret of child sexual abuse is finally revealed, Kayla was thrown into a series of events that initially left her feeling even more confused and out of control than before the disclosure. She describes the pilgrimage to Boston:

May 16, 2007 (age 16)

I sat in the middle, on a lawn chair as I drove toward my new hell. Mom was driving and humming a little tune along with the radio. Brian slept sitting straight up next to me.

Again I found myself thinking of him, of what I had done. I needed to talk to him. But how? The chair was uncomfortable, and I propped my feet on the moving truck's dashboard to try and compensate. She noticed my movement and automatically began to question.

"Hey, babe, how are you feeling?"

"How do you think, Mom? You're driving me to Boston, so I can live on my own with complete strangers to do a fucking sport. A sport I don't even want to fucking do. I hate it and you don't give a fuck—what else is new?"

The words left my throat and fresh tears began to sting the back of my eyes. I could tell I had hurt her feelings. Good. Serves her right for banishing me to hell.

"You think this is easy for any of us? You think I want you to move this far away?"

I cut her off before she could guilt me. "Yah, I do, Mom. I know you do because you're the one who's been trying to get me to move here for a year. All your little meetings with Jimmy Pedro. All the insistent hints . . . 'He's not good enough, Kay, you need to get away from him, Kay.' Well, congratulations, you got your wish, I'm gone. He's in jail. Did everything turn out the way you planned? I hope you're happy."

So began Kayla's journey to Boston after breaking her silence, a journey that threatened at times to again spin out of control as she dealt with feelings of sadness, shame, anger, and guilt following her disclosure and Daniel's arrest. Kayla wondered what control, if any, she would still have over the future direction of her life. Her confidences had been shattered, and she, like many such children, felt as if she no longer had a say in where she went, who she saw, and what adults and agencies would be involved in her life.

The effect of disclosure on the child, if not handled sensitively, can feel as traumatizing to the victim as the initial abuse. Families, as well, often talk about the total loss of privacy and control they feel following a sexual abuse revelation. Given this fact, it's critical for parents, educators, and involved child protection and legal professionals to pay attention to how best to guide children safely through the postdisclosure process, ensuring that they are given the information, choices, and personal respect that will ultimately make a difference to their degree of recovery.

A disclosure of child sexual abuse sets off a cascade of events, both internal and external. In many cases, victims can find themselves suddenly plunged into the legal system, with little understanding of what's happening to them, what will happen, and how to handle it all. The artificial sense of control that their silence may have provided them is now wrenched away, leaving them feeling unsafe in a new environment and suffering new forms of emotional upheaval. Chapter 4 helps you understand what you and your child might expect and offers advice for protecting your child from the collateral damage of seeing justice served.

Just as important—and necessary to address both simultaneously and going forward—are the long-term emotional effects of the abuse. The fact that the abuse has stopped and (in most cases) the victim is no longer in danger from the perpetrator does not mean the internal distress has ended. It's important to be alert for signs of ongoing—and sometimes temporarily worsening—symptoms, which we cover in Chapter 5, and often to obtain qualified professional help to ensure the best chances of recovery, the subject of Chapter 6. As we noted in the Introduction, we discuss postdisclosure information and advice over the span of these three chapters to make it manageable, but to be prepared for the immediate and later repercussions of disclosure, we suggest that all three chapters be read together.

4

Freedom with Its Own Chains
WHAT TO EXPECT AFTER DISCLOSURE

As Kayla's journey to Boston continued, she experienced firsthand the immediate fallout of her disclosure—repercussions all too common for children who are sexually abused:

> "Wow . . . How fast were you going, Brian?"
>
> Mom gives him a stern look, and I step over her and get out of the truck. The weight I've put on since after Senior Nationals is starting to take a toll on my body. Depression has always made me an emotional eater.
>
> But this time the depression stretches bigger than my stomach. I walk slowly toward the bathroom. A slight sweat breaks out on my skin. The people pumping gas are staring.
>
> Is it that obvious that I've lost my mind? Can you tell when a person has gone mad with grief? With guilt? I pick up the pace and put my head down.
>
> After Brian finishes pumping gas, Mom jumps in the driver's seat and Brian helps me back in the truck. He lifts me so gently, almost as if he's afraid I'll break. I don't blame him. Being around me causes everyone to walk on eggshells.
>
> I doze off again as the rain continues to pour, and this time I have a dream. I feel my body sweating, I'm trying to scream, but it won't come out. I'm frozen where I stand. Brian is shaking me

awake, and just like that, before the nightmare has even begun, it's over. He's saved me again.

I stare out the window for the remainder of the drive. Brian and Mom don't bother to try to get me to talk. I think they gave up on that about 2 hours ago. Brian periodically rubs my feet. And Mom rubs my hand between hers. I sneak a glance at her and I see the tears welling in her eyes. It doesn't even register in my mind. Nothing does anymore.

When we arrive, Mom and Brian unpack. I help a little. And just like that I'm on my way back to the mat for the first time in over a month . . .

If you're the parent of a child who has been sexually abused, disclosure (or discovery) feels like not just a tipping point but also a turning point. Once the abuse is brought out in the open, your son or daughter's victimization can now end and the perpetrator can be punished. Your child's safety, which you may have worried about for a long time, seems ensured.

Unfortunately, it's not that simple. The physical harm may have ended, but the psychological damage, discussed fully in Chapter 5, can plague a child well into adulthood. What is surprising to most people, however, is that victims can be, paradoxically, at their most vulnerable in some ways during the period *immediately* following disclosure or discovery. Anticipating this vulnerability is essential. In their understandable eagerness to stop the child abuser and prevent further harm to their child and to other children, parents and other adults often rush into decisions that can be damaging to the child they're trying to protect. Additionally, parents themselves often don't understand the legalities and protections that accompany a sexual abuse disclosure and so can be caught flat-footed when it comes to helping their child know what to anticipate next. Armed with knowledge, a parent can help guide him or her through the aftermath of this discovery.

When a child has disclosed being sexually assaulted (or it has been revealed otherwise), the child's retaining a sense of control over what happens next is paramount. A child who has been subjected to abuse has had to devise ways to manage powerful emotions like guilt and shame, as well as ways to deal with the cognitive dissonance of being harmed by someone who is supposed to be trustworthy—an authoritative or even loving adult. When the abuse is brought into the light of day, a chain of legal and other events is set in motion that disarms those protective defenses and wrests control from the child. *That is, unless parents and other adults charged with the child's protection stop and think, carefully considering how to proceed before taking hasty actions.*

That is the central message of this chapter: If you have just learned that your daughter or son has been a victim of child sexual abuse, resist the urge to rush into action. Read about the legal and related ramifications of disclosure in the pages that follow and carefully consider how to preserve your child's sense of control over what happens next. Also read Chapters 5 and 6 to become aware of how to address the lasting emotional effects of sexual abuse.

Children need to know what their choices are (if any) and need time to process what's happening. Kayla says it best:

> Looking back, there is so much I wish had been done differently in my case. I wish I didn't have to tell my story over and over again to different people. The prosecutor, the local police, the FBI, the victim witness advocate, etc. I wish I had been able to speak to them without my mother in the room. To have to talk about some of the most shameful aspects of my relationship with Daniel with my mother in the room sobbing was one of the hardest things I ever had to do. It was traumatizing to both of us in so many ways.
>
> I wish that the process had been a little bit slower. I know it took over a year and during that time there were many false starts and moments of doubt, and I know my mother wishes it had been faster, but I was very, very, very confused. And the only outlet I felt safe with was judo. Because my mother pushed so much and wanted justice so swiftly, it pushed us apart and pushed me further and further away from her. I wish family counseling had been offered. I wish that we had been able to deal with it together instead of us being on two different pages.
>
> Most of all I wish the adults and people in charge had stopped even briefly for a second to realize they were dealing with a very emotionally and mentally scarred child. I was confused, angry, and isolated much more because of the process.

In this diary entry, the distress Kayla was feeling at the time is palpable as she cooperates with law enforcement in getting a recorded admission of Daniel's victimization of her:

May 5, 2007 (age 16)

I talked to him last night and we got it all on tape. I talked to him for over an hour. And I lied and I lied, and I feel like shit now because of it. I mean he believed everything I said. And he told me he loved me and he missed me. And what was I supposed to do? I fell right back into my old ways. I told him I missed him and I loved him and it went right back to how it was and God it was just like old times. And the thing that kills me most is that I still think I really do love him and need him. And I don't know what to do. I mean he admitted to everything, and I cried so much I wanted to scream STOP they're recording you, but the words never escaped my mouth. And I told him I'd call him back today, and part of me meant it. I want to talk to him so bad. I want—no, I need—to hear that he's okay and that everything will be all right. I need him and I feel so out of control, and no one will listen.

Throughout this chapter and in Chapter 5, we offer advice for making the immediate aftermath of a disclosure easier on victims. For parents and other caregivers, it's essential to understand that the disclosure or discovery process itself can be traumatic for a child who has been abused, despite the relief that everyone naturally feels that the abuse has ended. If you did everything you could to reassure your child that she would have your support and protection, as advised in Chapter 3, and it was only after receiving these reassurances that your child disclosed being victimized, you have some sense of the internal struggles she has been undergoing while keeping the secret. To help your child start to make a lasting emotional recovery, you need to continue to offer the same types of support:

- Be willing to listen with empathy and support after your child has disclosed abuse to you.
- Consistently express your belief in what your child has told you.
- Be vigilant in ensuring that everyone involved in your child's care and in any legal proceedings is also supportive.
- Tell your child whom you need to or want to inform about the disclosure.

- Do your best to allow your child time to process the emotional fallout from the initial disclosure before any further loss of anonymity and privacy.

- Help your child feel safe from the abuser by informing the child of when and how the perpetrator will be apprised of the disclosure and how the disclosure will likely affect his personal life, employment, and legal status.

In the box below, Kayla offers her own wisdom about what kinds of help she would have liked to receive from the justice system.

In keeping with Kayla's advice about how to improve the judicial process (see the box below), it's encouraging to see that progress is being made. Massachusetts, where we work, now uses a Sexual Assault Intervention Network (S.A.I.N.) interview as part of a multidisciplinary approach to child abuse that allows all the agencies involved to coordinate their efforts, investigate simultaneously, and conduct a single interview. These agencies include the district attorney's office, the Department of Children and Families, and law enforcement.

KAYLA'S SUGGESTIONS FOR MAKING THE JUSTICE-SEEKING PROCESS EASIER ON KIDS

- One interviewer, at one time, with expert interviewers and all others in a separate room to watch through a screen or window (police, prosecutors, doctors, etc., in a separate room, but all watching), with the child having the ability to ask the interviewer specific questions should they arise during the process.
- Family counseling.
- Material on others who have been through this process (such as this book or other stories of survivors who are willing to share).
- Court-ordered therapy for the victims. Victims or their parents may not always know they need help, but they do, and the court should be held accountable for making sure the child gets adequate help.
- Mandatory weekly updates from the prosecution on how the case is proceeding and a very clear-cut, understandable account of what steps are being taken (many times in my case I had no idea of whether we were going to court, or Daniel was pleading out, or what charges were being filed, etc.)

THE LOSS OF ANONYMITY

With the revelation of sexual abuse, the child loses the anonymity she has relied on to manage some of the powerful emotions, particularly guilt and shame, which typically increase as the abuse continues. With disclosure, children can feel distressingly exposed, with their feelings of guilt and shame continuing to escalate and persisting long after the abuse has ended. (You'll find help with handling these distressing symptoms in Chapter 5 and information on how different types of therapy address them in Chapter 6.) As Kayla described at the beginning of this chapter, she felt that even strangers at the gas station on the way to Boston somehow knew of her abuse by Daniel. Anonymity, ironically, also allows victims to continue to "enjoy" the benefits of the relationship with an individual who commonly holds a great deal of power in their lives and whom they have tried to see as appropriate, rather than abusive, in his attentions. Unless parents assure them that those benefits will be provided in other ways, this loss can feel like a blow too. Disclosure can feel like a form of freedom that comes with its own chains.

In the aftermath of disclosure children fear this loss of anonymity and often try to petition the person to whom they've disclosed not to let anyone else know about their revelation. As noted in Chapter 3, sometimes children attempt tentative disclosures to try to elicit what will happen if they break the silence, such as asking indirectly about what would happen to their anonymity and their confidences "if someone my age tells someone that they are being abused." Knowing the answers to such questions can prepare you to help an abused child and minimize her distress during the postdisclosure process. That's why a big part of this chapter is devoted to explaining the legal and other ramifications of disclosure. But you also need to be aware that the mere event of disclosure (or discovery) changes the landscape for a child who has been keeping this secret for so long, and it changes the child's internal landscape too. Even before any legalities enter the picture, you may see signs of increasing distress, especially shame and guilt, as the child faces the possibility that, now that one person knows about what has been happening to her, many others may end up knowing too. Suddenly the one area over which she had control—keeping the secret—has been lost to her. She may ask for repeated reassurances that the story will go no further or show what might seem like bizarre concern for the welfare of her abuser. These expressions of distress flow mainly from the shame and guilt that these children feel about having "allowed" themselves to be abused. Parents and other caring adults need to express support and compassion, but also tell the truth about who will likely end up knowing something about the child's story. We can't emphasize enough how important maintaining a sense of control is to a child who is emerging from the nightmare of abuse.

When talking to an abused child after disclosure,

Instead of saying . . .	Say . . .
"I won't tell anyone."	"I'm not sure yet who else will need to know what happened to you, but my only concern is your safety and well-being, and I will check into the mandated reporting requirements and let you know who I do need to notify about this."
"I am sure the police won't have to know."	"I will check with child protective services if we need to report to them and ask about whether the police will have to be notified."
"The police know what's best, so just give them the information that they ask you about."	"I understand how private this has been and that you are unsure about what you want to see happen to X; I will try to make sure that you're not pressured into anything and understand all of your options."
"I can't believe you'd care what happens to X [the abuser], now that we know he has hurt other people!"	"I don't know what will happen to X, and it may not be entirely in our control, but try to hang onto the truth that you are not responsible for any harm that comes to him."
"This is really hard for me too; I really need to talk to my friends/my family, etc."	"I understand that your privacy around this is most important, and I also could use someone to talk to. Is there anyone else that you feel comfortable with my sharing this with? If not, I will find a therapist who specializes in this to talk to."

Children subjected to sexual abuse understandably do not want their identity and abuse disclosed to people beyond their initial confidants until they are ready for wider disclosure, and depending on who this initial confidant is, they may have more or less time to accommodate to whatever loss of privacy is inevitable. Often children believe they are telling someone about their abuse in confidence, only to feel shocked and betrayed when the person they disclose to turns out to have an obligation, either mandated (as with licensed professionals like therapists and teachers) or based on personal beliefs about what the child needs, to report the abuse to others.

For a majority of child victims, disclosing is a confusing process, and they need the chance to understand what will happen step by step, including all of their options, up to and including what might or might not happen to the alleged perpetrator if they do or don't pursue criminal charges. Having the chance to talk through all of the emotional and practical consequences of the options available to them is critical to their ongoing recovery, and a knowledgeable professional can be very helpful here. In some cases the youth will be provided with a victim witness advocate by the office of the district attorney who is prosecuting the case, but having him or her see a mental health professional for ongoing therapy can often ease the long-term aftereffects of abuse, as described in Chapter 6. Again, we strongly recommend reading through everything in Chapters 4–6 if you're concerned about a youth who may be reaching the tipping point or has just disclosed sexual abuse, because the material in all three chapters is relevant simultaneously.

WHAT PARENTS AND CAREGIVERS NEED TO KNOW

To be most helpful in the immediate aftermath of a disclosure, parents, and really all adults, must be well informed about the range of accepted formal and informal responses to the revelation of abuse and how to keep this process as supportive and compassionate as possible for the child. Part of this necessary education includes understanding issues such as age of consent, mandated reporting requirements, and what to expect from child welfare and law enforcement agencies. Professionals and paraprofessionals who work with children now have this information at hand for the state they practice in as part of their

required training. Parents and caregivers, however, often find themselves completely in the dark when they are thrust into a situation in
which they need to help a child know his options, while maintaining
as much of a sense of dignity and control as possible throughout the
process.

Since this book does not claim to give legal advice and the laws
pertaining to child sexual abuse vary from state to state, this chapter presents an overview of general principles, with a focus on how
the application of these laws can affect your child's psychological
health after disclosure. (More specific information is provided in the
Resources section at the back of this book.)

Understanding how the entire process works in your locality may
take some time. You may have to ask the authorities lots of questions,
do your own research, and be firm about your desire to protect your
child's welfare above all else. Until you feel you know (almost) exactly
what will happen, remain honest with your child that you are not
sure of the whole process but that you're going to take things slowly
and do your best to shield her from unanticipated events that she
finds distressing. At the same time, take every opportunity to state to
authorities that your child's well-being is your number-one priority.
Never hesitate to ask individual authorities how they plan to protect
your child's welfare while following the law. Everyone wants justice to
be served in the face of the heinous act of child sexual abuse, but no
child should suffer further to achieve that goal.

Age of Consent Repercussions

Many people are not aware that every state in America, along with
most countries around the world, has a formal *age of consent* that
defines the age at which a child is considered legally competent to
engage in a sexual relationship with someone above that age. The dis-
tinctive characteristic of the age of consent laws in most jurisdictions
is that persons below the minimum age of consent are considered
the victims, and the older persons with whom they have sex are considered perpetrators. In other words, what we're calling child sexual
abuse can legally be a crime committed by, say, an 18-year-old having
sex with a 17-year-old. That the older teen may be considered a perpetrator in the eyes of the law can be very difficult for parents to accept
and is very important for teenagers to understand. In the individual
states, the age of consent is somewhere between 16 and 18, but other

factors may also be relevant. For example, the age of consent may differ within a state for the purposes of civil versus criminal law, and the age of consent may vary if the older person is in a position of authority. More details are given on page 108. Knowing these facts for your specific state and talking with your teen about them can go a long way toward helping to keep children of all ages from being harmed, and in some cases from harming one another.

In Kayla's case, there was no doubt that she had not reached the age of consent when sexual contact with Daniel began or for most of the time it continued (generally speaking, the age of consent in Ohio, where she lived, is 16, although, as we'll see, the fact that the abuse occurred outside of Ohio as well had further legal repercussions). In other cases the line seems blurrier, since young teenagers are often sexually active, but the law sees it clearly, and charges of statutory rape can be brought when, for example, a 14-year-old high school freshman consents to sexual contact with a 17-year-old junior or senior. That does not mean that charges will

> Make sure your children are familiar with the age of consent in your state so they know there can be serious legal repercussions for having any sexual contact with someone under that age.

always be brought; the local authorities have some discretion here. But it does mean that it's possible. Here again, for parents who may have children of various ages, it is essential to educate every teen to know the age when he becomes an adult in the eyes of the law so that he appreciates the potential repercussions of having any form of sexual relations with someone below that age.

Mandated Reporting Rules

Every state in the United States, as well as many countries around the world, has developed a system of child welfare laws and sanctions geared toward protecting children under a specific age from neglect and abuse of various kinds by an adult; this includes sexual abuse. In Massachusetts, for example, the age of consent is 16. This means that in Massachusetts—as in every other state—Kayla's being touched inappropriately at age 12 by an adult who at that time was 24 constituted abuse. An adult who learns of such abuse needs to know what the *reporting obligations* are for notifying the local child welfare authorities.

Most mandated reporting requirements established by state law apply to those acting in a professional capacity with regard to the abused child. This means that a doctor, teacher, therapist, and any other adult who operates in a supervisory role with children must report suspected or confirmed child abuse to the local authorities. For a minor child, the agency involved is child protective services, which usually has a toll-free hotline available for reporting. If abuse is reported directly to the police, the police department will notify the child welfare agency if the child is under 18. If the child is older than 18 at the time of the report, the report will go directly to the police rather than being screened for child welfare involvement (as occurs for all abuse and neglect reports by a child under age 18). In this case the focus will be on the criminal aspect of the case and child welfare will not get involved—unless there are other minor children in the home or the suspected person is in a job like teacher or coach, supervising minor children. It does not necessarily mean that a child's friend (Brian) or a parent (Kayla's mother) is required to report the abuse (although they may be, depending on the age of the friend and also the state where the abuse occurs).

> Most of the individuals mandated by law to report child abuse are professionals involved in their care, from doctors to teachers, therapists, and others.

THE CHILD ABUSE PREVENTION AND TREATMENT ACT

The key federal legislation addressing child abuse and neglect in the United States is the Child Abuse Prevention and Treatment Act (CAPTA), originally enacted in 1974 (*www.childwelfare.gov*). CAPTA is the act that originally established the national Office of Child Abuse and Neglect, which sets forth a minimum definition of child abuse and neglect; however, specific child protection laws are established and governed by state statutes and regulations.

The mandated reporting obligation for child abuse and neglect, like the age of consent, is defined by each of the 50 states. These state-mandated reporting laws indicate whether you are required by law to report a disclosure of child abuse to others and, if so, specifically to whom. Knowing the reporting requirements ahead of time will help you provide accurate information to any child who is considering disclosure and help the child reveal her secret.

These individuals typically have a designated reporting obligation:

- Social workers
- Teachers, principals, and other school personnel
- Physicians, nurses, and other health care workers
- Counselors, therapists, and other mental health professionals
- Child care providers
- Law enforcement officers

Some states, however, require *anyone* who suspects a child is being abused to report it. If you reside in one of those states, you would be required, for example, to report on a neighbor that you suspect of abuse or face potential criminal penalties yourself. As of 2017, these states are Delaware, Florida, Idaho, Indiana, Kentucky, Maryland, Mississippi, Nebraska, New Hampshire, New Jersey, New Mexico, North Carolina, Oklahoma, Rhode Island, Tennessee, Texas, Utah, and Wyoming, along with Puerto Rico. This list could be longer by the time you read this book. Critical information about your own state's rules is available from *www.childwelfare.gov/pubPDFs/manda.pdf.* Current statute information for a particular state is available from *www.childwelfare.gov/topics/ systemwide/laws-policies/state.*

> In 18 states *every* citizen is mandated to report child abuse.

While mandatory reporting is just that, *mandatory,* the adult's job is not made easier by compelling a child or teen to reveal more specifics about the abuse than he or she is ready to; rather it's important that the adult and child work collaboratively and carefully to consider the child's fears and together consider the benefits to the child of fully disclosing. The reporting obligation does not extend to friends if they are not yet adults themselves and may not apply to members of the clergy; but again, depending on what state you live in, family, older peers, and clergy may all have a mandated reporting responsibility. A clergy member's obligation to report depends, for example, on the person's specific role with regard to the child or teen, and even the exception for spiritual counseling has recently changed in many states, making it essential to let your child or a youth you are talking with know exactly who is mandated to report abuse and how it should be handled according to the *current* law in your state. Only in this way can both you and your child be prepared to jointly negotiate the precarious period of time following child abuse revelations.

In our clinical practices a majority of youngsters want to know, as the first step in considering disclosure, what we will do with the information they provide. If your child asks you a leading question like "What would happen if one of my friends told someone that she was being hurt?" you have an opportunity—*if* you've informed yourself of the mandated reporting laws in your state—to tell her whether she could disclose to a parent anonymously and what the reporting consequences would be of talking to someone like a teacher. Many older adolescents in particular are looking to get help in ending an abusive situation without identifying their perpetrator, which is sometimes possible, as in instances when the abuse is happening elsewhere (in another state) or a now-older child wants to discuss ways of removing himself entirely from a home situation where he was abused in the more distant past. Remember as well that the mandated reporting responsibility applies to individuals under 18 years of age.

Again, an opening to talk about reporting is an even more important opportunity to assure your child that you will be there to protect her and, above all, that you will help her stay informed and in as much control over the process of disclosure as possible. We delve into this subject in more depth in Chapter 5, but the point now is that control is paramount to children who have been sexually abused, and anything you can do from the start to show that you will respect the child's feelings, within the law, will support the process of disclosure and ensuing recovery.

What Happens after Child Sexual Abuse Is Reported?

Once child protective services receives a mandated report of child sexual abuse, the agency will take the following steps:

- *Screen out the initial report* as not meeting the criteria for abuse or neglect; this happens when the child is no longer living with a specific adult, the alleged abuse happened in the distant past but was just discovered, or the abuse reported is emotional or physical but of a "minor" nature. Reports being screened out are not uncommon because mandated reporting laws require that any report by a child or suspicion of abuse is initially reported.

- *Screen in the initial report for further evaluation,* which involves an evaluation that is conducted over a period of days or weeks, depending on the nature of the report and specific state-level guidelines. At the end of the evaluation period the report of abuse is either *supported or unsupported.*

- *Act on supported allegations.* In most states the child and family will be assigned a social worker to monitor their well-being and safety in the home for some period of time. In cases of support the alleged perpetrator will also be entered into the state database as having a substantiated abuse or neglect report on file.

In Kayla's case, the lack of knowledge about Ohio's child protection statutes and related criminal law led to Kayla's immediately facing unexpected repercussions from family and outside agencies:

When I talked to Brian, it was nowhere in my mind how he would react or who he would tell. Before I could think straight he was insisting that I call my mother, who was on a plane flying home, and all I remember is leaving her a message on her voice mail, although the terror I was gripped with overran any real sense of the words I was saying, except to know that these words were certain to seal my own fate along with Daniel's.

Neither can I now remember when and how I found out that my mother had, upon hearing my revelation on her phone, taken a bat and smashed up not only Daniel's car but also some of the windows of his house. She also called the police, although, again, I cannot say when I found this out or how much time passed before Brian and I arrived home.

Many people believe it is in the child's best interest to report abuse, if for no other reason than to make sure the perpetrator is punished and does not victimize another child. In this regard Kayla's experience is a cautionary tale, not against reporting Daniel's crimes but against doing so before a child has the opportunity to anticipate what might happen and what her options are. It's important to know your state's mandated reporting laws because if those laws do *not* mandate reporting abuse that is revealed to you, then you have the option of taking time to think—and to help your child process what might happen. You may want to wait even if your every instinct tells you to rush to the authorities and ensure that justice is done. In fact, even when reporting *is* mandated, if you understand the legal process we've described, you can explain it to your child so she has time to feel some measure of control.

In Kayla's case the time to process her ordeal was lost as she was taken almost immediately to the local police station after her mother had already lodged a complaint against Daniel for sexual assault. To this day the memory is accompanied by confusion and feelings of heightened distress:

Nor can I tell you exactly when I went to the police station or who was there when I first went in to be questioned. I do remember vividly, however, that they asked me to make out a list of the "sexual encounters" I had had with Daniel.

I remember it being the worst day of my life, and that the process lasted several exhausting hours, and that I hated every single person in that room for making me write down my guilt and my secrets for them to pass around and share.

I was angry, exhausted, scared, alone, and very very confused as to whose fault all of this was. I wasn't angry with Daniel. I was angry with the police, I was angry at my mother, I was angry at everyone for making me do this.

And I have kept a copy of that horrible, handwritten list of offenses written on lined notebook paper with my 16-year-old scribbles in the margins. A list that to others confirmed that Daniel was a child molester and made me feel like a horrible and guilty person, a person who was betraying her best friend.

What About the Police and Criminal Charges?

Even when a parent chooses not to go directly to the police as Kayla's mother did, if the parent or another adult has informed a local child protective services agency or a hotline about the abuse, and the report is eventually supported, the local child abuse and neglect office will report the abuse to the legal authorities. Children who are sexually abused and their families are often unaware that child welfare agencies that receive a report of disclosed or suspected abuse frequently have their own obligation to inform law enforcement that abuse or neglect rising to the level of a crime has likely been committed against a minor child.

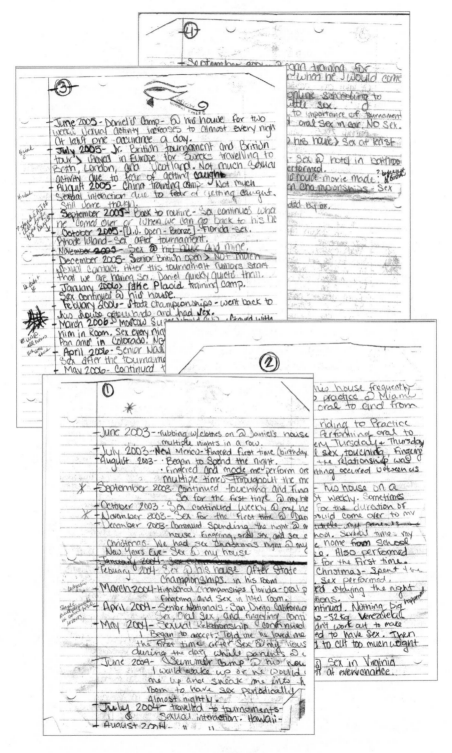

④

- September 2006 - Began training for
  when he would come
- online schooling to
  ...ttle sex.
- to importance of tournament
  oral sex in ear. NO Sex.
- his house.) sex at least
- Sex @ hotel in bathtub...
  performed.
- house movie made: ? ...
  n championships - Sex
  ...ded by me.

③

- June 2005 - Daniel's Camp- @ his house for two weeks. Sexual activity increases to almost every night. At least one occurance a day.
- July 2005- Jr. British tournament and British tour. Played in Europe for 3 weeks travelling to Bath, London, and Scotland. Not much sexual activity due to fear of getting caught.
- August 2005- China training camp- Not much sexual interaction due to fear of getting caught. Still some though.
- September 2005- back to routine- Sex continues when he comes over or when we can go back to his ho...
- October 2005- [U.S. open - Bronze] -Florida- sex. Rhode Island- Sex after tournament.
- November 2005- Sex @ his house and mine.
- December 2005- Senior British open > NOT much sexual contact. After this tournament rumors start that we are having sex. Daniel quickly quiets them.
- January 2006- Lake Placid training camp. Sex continued @ his house.
- February 2006- State championships- went back to his house afterwards and had sex.
- March 2006- Moscow ... Played with him in room. Sex every night ... Pan am? in Colorado. NG...
- April 2006- Senior Nat... Sex after the tournament...
- May 2006- Continued ...

②

his house frequently
practice @ Miami
oral to and from

riding to practice
Performing oral to
every Tuesday + Thursday
l sex, touching, fingering
the relationship was
...thing occured between us

his house on a
t weekly. Sometimes
for the duration of
ould come over to my
ttle my parents
ool. Several time - my
e home from school
e. Also performed
for the first time.
Christmas- spent the
sex performed.
staying the night
tions.
ntinued. Nothing big
s - 52 kg Venezuela?
dn't work out to make
ed to have sex. Then
to cut too much weight

Sex in Virginia
at every chance.

①

*

- June 2003- rubbing w/clothes on @ Daniel's house multiple nights in a row.
- July 2003- New Mexico- Fingered first time (birthday
- August 2003- - Began to spend the night.
  - Fingered and made me perform ora...
    multiple times throughout the mo...
- September 2003- Continued touching and fing... Sex for the first time @ my ho...
- October 2003- Sex continued weekly @ my ho...
- November 2003- Sex for the first time @ Dan...
- December 2003- Continued spending the night @ h... house. Fingering, oral sex, and sex c... Christmas- We had sex Christmas night @ my... New Years Eve- Sex @ my house
- January 2004-
- February 2004- Sex @ his house after State championships. in his room.
- March 2004- Highschool championships Florida- oral s... Fingering and Sex in hotel room.
- April 2004- Senior Nationals- San Diego California... Sex, oral sex, and fingering conti...
- May 2004- Sexual Relationship continued. I began to accept. Told me he loved me the first time after sex @ my ... during the day while parents ...
- June 2004- Summer Camp @ his hou... I would wake up or he would... me up and sneak me into h... room to have sex periodically. Almost nightly.
- July 2004- travelled to tournaments- Sexual interaction. Hawaii...
- August 2004- '' ''

What is considered criminal, as explained earlier, varies by state. Not only is it determined at first by the age of consent, but also by factors, such as the type of sexual act, the gender of the participants, and other restrictions defined as abuses of a *position of trust*. For most purposes a *position of trust* includes parents, anyone acting in the place of parents and charged with the parent's rights and duties, or anyone charged with the health, education, and welfare of and supervision of a child. Crimes against children committed by someone in a position of trust are taken more seriously. The significance of the concept of *position of trust* is that, even if a child is older than the state's age of consent, if she is a minor (under age 18), she can still be considered virtually powerless to consent to sexual contact with someone who has some form of authority over her (a teacher or clergy member, for example), and the person in a position of trust can therefore be charged with criminal sexual abuse of a child. Some jurisdictions include exceptions for minors engaged in sexual acts with each other, rather than using a single age. Also, the specific legal charges resulting from a violation of these child protection laws can range from a misdemeanor, such as corruption of a minor, to what is more commonly known as statutory rape, which is considered equivalent to rape, in both severity and sentencing.

> What is considered criminal varies by state, but can depend in part on whether the alleged abuser occupied a position of trust—was charged with the health, education, welfare, and supervision of the child—at the time of the abuse.

Only by knowing the range of potential outcomes following the discovery of sexual abuse is it possible to *guide a child* effectively through this process, helping him to understand the limits of his rights and privileges. Would your child feel differently about pressing charges if the charge were a misdemeanor versus a felony that came with a potentially long sentence—as it did for Daniel? Would your 17-year-old feel like a contributor to her sexual abuse because she no longer considers herself a child? The laws (and the best interests of the child) might not allow the affected youth or parents to make many choices about the legal ramifications of a disclosure, but considering these issues can help everyone anticipate the emotional impact on the youth and exert every possible effort to afford her some sense of control and to protect her well-being. These issues are addressed in Chapter 5.

The Importance of the Wishes of the Victim and Family

In reality, enforcement practices involving age-of-consent laws vary widely depending on many factors, the most important of which should be, and often is, the wishes of the victim and their family. To put it simply, when police and prosecutors have discretion over what charge they can choose to bring in a certain situation, the wishes of the victim need to be made paramount if at all possible. For example, in a case in which one adult hurts multiple children, no one individual child will be able to stop the prosecution, and each one may be subpoenaed to testify even if reluctant. However, in cases like Kayla's, where there are no other known victims, it is largely up to the victim and her parents to decide what, if any, charges will be pursued.

Unfortunately, it is often in the throes of anger at the perpetrator at first hearing the disclosure that parents act directly to file a criminal complaint, without pausing to take into account how those actions may affect their child, both in the shorter and longer term. When there has been an enduring relationship between the victim and the abuser, the victim often feels torn about both the publicity and punishment that may accompany court proceedings. Even in cases with minor children, when an effort is made to hide the identity of the victim in court records, the local community and press often find out what is happening and reveal details about the participants. This occurred when Daniel was first arrested. His local prominence as a coach and common knowledge of the students he worked with led to rampant and sometimes hurtful speculations about Kayla's identity, which at the time only added to her confusion and self-blame.

Kayla looks back to the point, when she had been in Boston for only a few months, when, she says, already so much had happened:

At an event in Florida a well-known senior male judoka called my room. I had known his new girlfriend, a Cuban judoka, when I lived in Ohio, and I said hello to her. She must have misunderstood my skittish body language and darting eye contact as rude because when I got up to my room her boyfriend called.

"Hello," I said.

"Is this Kayla?" said a male voice that I didn't recognize.

"Yes," I said.

"What did you say to Maria?"

"I'm sorry?" I said, confused.

"What did you say to her? Huh?" he said, angrier now.

"I said hello. I don't know what else you're talking about," I said, getting nervous now.

"You are just Daniel's whore, you know that? You know that everyone knows you fucked Daniel, right?" he says and then hangs up on me.

My mom comes back to the room to find me in tears. It's not much, but when you are 16 and trying to put your life back together, a small moment like that can feel like a mountain.

Online chat rooms make it worse. Grown men and women discussing whether or not I was of legal age when things began. Discussing if I "wanted it" or not. Talking about my private personal life right there for anyone to read.

Many said they would kill Daniel if it was their child. Many said I was old enough to know what I was doing. Particular members of the judo forum loved getting into the grit of it and discussing what is legal and what's not in which state and so on. As the case developed and the charges were pressed, many would jump online to give their two cents. When Daniel finally pled guilty, the forum eventually fizzled out. There was nothing left to discuss, except whether or not I would stick around or become anything.

But it never stopped me from getting on and checking what people were saying. I would check in periodically for years down the line until finally the thread could no longer be found. Always wondering who belonged to which screen name. I have no doubt that they would never say to my face what was said online in those forums about my honesty, my integrity. If I was telling the truth or just seeking attention.

To this day I attend judo events and I see that man that called my room. He has never apologized.

To this day I attend judo events and I wonder if the person who said that 12 is old enough to know better is in the room. Or if the person who said I only wanted attention is standing in line waiting for my autograph. Or if the one who said I'd never make it has a picture with me hanging in their dojo. I was young and scared and in the worst moments of my life. And having that kind of attention and gossip surround me made it ten times worse. But it also made me stronger. And now I am not a young scared girl. I am a strong, confident woman who's not afraid to tell people that what you say DOES affect people. Sometimes more than you know. So be careful.

*You never know what people are battling, and you never know who
you may help. With a kind word or a smile, it can go a long way in
making someone's journey that much better. And just to clear the
record—I was not old enough. It was NOT my fault. I did NOT quit.
And I never will.*

Although prosecution of child sexual abuse often requires the
victim to be willing and able to testify to secure a conviction, when
the perpetrator is in a position of power over other minor children the
victim often experiences a great deal of pressure to press charges and
provide testimony for the benefit of others who might be harmed if the
alleged abuser remains free. These competing pressures on a young
child can lead to her feeling "traumatized again" in the short run, feeling helpless and coerced into a decision to press charges without having her personal wishes and feelings taken fully into account. Kayla
had to face the painful emotional and practical reality that Daniel's
fate lay largely in her hands and that her statements could send him
to prison. Because of his status and notoriety as a coach, and the clear
manner in which Daniel had used this role to gain access to his victim,
both the police and Kayla's parents exerted pressure on Kayla to press
criminal charges and prosecute Daniel to the full extent of the law.

Looking back, Kayla says:

*I had a victim witness advocate, and I got pamphlets about
victim rights. But I never felt as if there was a choice about prosecuting him. Definitely not. The prosecutor, the FBI, the victim witness advocate, my parents, everyone was, like, "He could do this to
someone else." What I suggest parents say to kids now is: "I know
you feel helpless. I know you feel scared. I know you are feeling empty
and alone. But I promise you—it will get better. And the first step
has already been taken. You have been so brave and so strong. You
have spoken up and said something. And we believe you. Now you
must believe and trust that I and the authorities are going to do the
right thing. And the right thing is to make sure that X never hurts
anyone else again. I know it's hard, but I want you to trust me. And
I want you to help me. And I want to help you. I'll be with you every
step of the way."*

Before she had time to consider or reconsider, Kayla was con-
fronted with not only local but also state and federal authorities as

it became apparent that the crimes committed against her had been perpetrated both on national and international soil during their travels to competitions. Kayla's distress and confusion over the largely unanticipated, and at the time largely unwanted, consequences of her disclosure are evident in writings from the period immediately following Daniel's arrest, as she began to contemplate the likely impact of her revelations on Daniel.

In one excerpt she describes the series of events following her disclosure to Brian and how they had changed just about everything in her life and left her feeling traumatized a second time:

> I let my body return to numbness. It was easier this way. To not think, feel, or do anything. I remember when I first told, I would sit in my room for hours. Just lay there. And I would sleep 14 hours a night. My body so exhausted with depression. My muscles stiff from lack of use and the weight of the guilt I was carrying.
>
> The police had me and my mom call him and get a recorded confession. When he was talking to my mom, she was crying and telling Daniel that she couldn't put me through this; that if he just told she would drop the charges.
>
> What hurt the most was I knew that she was acting. She lied and said she didn't want to put me through this, but she didn't even seem to care. She was so worked up on her own revenge that she threw me to the wolves. The police also seemed to just want revenge; they did not want to really hear from me and only cared that I write down the facts, even though the facts don't really tell the whole story . . .
>
> I was not either angry or sad—I just didn't care, and that scared me. But I was compliant, so I told the police what they wanted to know. And then Daniel was arrested and released on bail and there was a restraining order hearing and the day of the restraining order hearing my mom packed me up and moved me to Boston.
>
> That was the longest time I ever went without judo, without him.

Effects on the Family

It's also important to consider here how the unanticipated consequences of sexual abuse disclosures can affect not only the victim but also the victim's family. After Daniel was quickly released on bail pending his court case, Kayla and her family were left to contend with the rumor mill churning in the small world of Ohio judo, which at times *blamed the victim* for pressing charges against a highly esteemed and well-known local sports figure and also questioned how the abuse had gone unnoticed for so long by Kayla's family. Kayla's mother hoped that moving her daughter to Boston would shield Kayla, at least in part, from the daily reminders of the trauma and allow her to continue to train in the sport she had devoted herself to since the age of 8. But it was hard on her younger brother and sister, as Kayla's mother describes:

> "They didn't know what was happening, only that you were gone. And that affected them most. They missed you. They missed their big sister. What impacted them was you moving away. Your sister started acting out and hanging with the wrong people. We were so focused on you, though, that I let a lot of that go by and didn't take appropriate action and it affected her later in life. I don't feel as if what happened to our family affected my decisions about court, though. Not at all. What impacted my decision was that you didn't want to live. You needed to do your sport. You needed a reason to wake up."

Kayla says she believes it was the lack of any ongoing dialogue and support that "tore my family apart," as her sister was only 12 and her brother 8 when Kayla essentially disappeared, unfortunately, leaving everyone in Ohio to reconstruct their own lives after the abuse was revealed.

WHAT'S NEXT?

As we've previously stated, if your child's abuse has been determined to meet the criteria established for child abuse and neglect in your state, it will be accepted for an investigation or assessment. In general, cases that involve physical or sexual abuse or possible criminal conduct are investigated by a law enforcement agency, while other types of maltreatment are referred for family assessments that are conducted primarily by the child protective services agency. More and more, states are using a team-assessment approach, typically involving representatives from child protective services, law enforcement, and prosecutors' offices, who work together to reduce the negative impact on child victims of having to undergo multiple interviews with different personnel.

The primary purpose of an investigation or assessment done by child protective services or law enforcement is to establish whether the allegation of abuse or neglect is supportable and, if it is, to make sure that the child is protected going forward. It is important to understand that the focus is on determining the nature, extent, and cause of the abuse or neglect and identifying the person responsible for the maltreatment. The focus is not on specifically evaluating the mental and emotional well-being of the child, which needs to be addressed as well (see Chapter 6).

Elements of an investigation may include:

- A visit to the child's home.
- An interview of the child victim.
- Interviews or observation of other children living in the child's home.
- An evaluation of the home environment.
- Interviews with the child's parents, caregivers, or other adults residing in the child's home.
- Checks of criminal records and central registry records for the alleged perpetrator.
- A referral for medical and mental health evaluations.

Assessment interviews that take place following a complaint to a state agency need to be differentiated from the evaluations done by mental health professionals to assess whether, and what kind of, ongoing therapy may be indicated. If your child has just disclosed sexual abuse to you, your first instinct may be to consult your pediatrician or another trusted health care provider. Just understand that this consultation is no substitute for dealing with child protective services or the legal system, and remember that in every state health care professionals, such as physicians and nurse practitioners, have a mandated reporting obligation in cases involving childhood abuse and neglect.

WORSENING DISTRESS
FOLLOWING DISCLOSURE

Early in this chapter we mentioned that parents may very well notice an increase in an abused child's distress right after disclosure. The events just described illustrate this phenomenon. We hear repeatedly in our work with children subjected to this abuse and their families that the initial period after disclosure is traumatic for the child and family alike. This is, after all, when the child typically gives her first statements and interviews to law enforcement and/or child protection personnel, requiring her to relive the details of her abuse in the presence of strangers. Going through this process and making decisions about whether to formally prosecute the offender is a complicated and challenging ordeal, made only worse when youth are not helped to understand and anticipate the likely events that will follow and what decisions they will generally be required to make. Sometimes, if the perpetrator is a family member, victimized youth can additionally face either being taken out of their own home or, alternatively, having the offender barred from having contact with any other minor children in the family. All of these repercussions, which affect the youth's privacy and relationships with her family, friends, community, and even the perpetrator, are a source of tremendous emotional upheaval for him or her.

Kayla remembers feeling alone and misunderstood immediately following her disclosure to Brian, turning again to her journal to express her confusion and distress, which had not abated and perhaps had worsened since she revealed her abuse:

May 18, 2007 (age 16)

Dear God,

Well, it's been a while, and a lot has changed in a month. The secret's out. The secret that I couldn't even write to you about.

Everyone knows I had sex with Daniel. I told the truth. I told them it was a relationship and I consented.

My mom is filing charges. I'm going along with it, but I know he doesn't deserve it. I keep telling myself that I knew what was going on and I was in control of myself.

I know Daniel is being punished for my sins. I'm the one that should go to jail. I know I deserve to go to hell.

God, please forgive me. Please help me. So many emotions going through me.

Everything I see I see his reflection. Everything I think I hear his voice. Everything I do I hear his reactions. He's stuck in my head and I can't get him out.

God, please help me. When I saw him in court on Tuesday, it was like my whole world came crashing down and my resolution to end this hasn't been the same since.

I will say that Brian has been there for me 100%. Knowing he's there for me and by my side makes me so grateful. It also makes it worse.

Everyone sees me as a victim, but you and I know the truth. I am nothing but a whore. A manipulative whore that cares only about herself.

Please God, help me.

Love Always,
Kayla

This entry captures the complicated reactions that often accompany disclosure when a criminal complaint or arrest quickly follows the initial revelation. We noted earlier that you may be surprised to hear your child express anxiety over what will happen to the abuser now that the truth is out. Although their belief is counterintuitive, victims often feel responsible for their abuser's fate, having intended only to end the abuse and not yet sure that the perpetrator deserves the full force of public condemnation and potential imprisonment. And after what has often been years of involvement, the sea change that follows both disclosure and the consequent reporting repercussions can challenge the victim's core sense of identity and control. We talk more about such reactions in Chapter 5 and how various therapies can help abused children handle them in Chapter 6.

Considering the Burden of Serving as a Witness

Often it's difficult for law enforcement to actually go to trial against a child sexual abuse perpetrator without the cooperation and assistance of the victim. This is especially true for adolescent victims, who are often disclosing abuse that has taken place over a significant period of time in the past and for which there may be no fresh physical or corroborating evidence. While the abuse of younger children may be discovered or interrupted by an adult and the child can be immediately examined for forensic evidence of the abuse, this approach is generally not possible for the preteen or teen victim, whose narrative about what happened may be all the authorities have to go on. This circumstance makes it inordinately challenging for older victims to evaluate what they are prepared to say to law enforcement personnel and to fully understand the pros and cons of filing a criminal complaint. Clearly they need support from parents and professionals to manage this process.

In most jurisdictions, there are specific staff attached to the district attorney's office, commonly referred to as victim witness advocates, whose job it is to help conduct interviews with the victim and serve as liaisons to police, families, and the court, with the goal of helping a victim understand the range of potential charges that might be brought, what the court process entails, and what are the victim's rights and risks as a central witness in a sexual abuse prosecution. As with all other aspects of the disclosure process, however, the more information and resources a victim and her parents have, the better they fare emotionally, as they collectively face making critical decisions in the criminal justice process. All too often not only the child but the nonoffending adults in the child's life can feel blamed and stigmatized once abuse has been made public, and this only further heightens the victim's distress during what is already a difficult time.

For Kayla, the decision to prosecute Daniel and commit to all that followed in the courts went on over quite some time as she, like so many other children who've experienced abuse, tried valiantly to pick up the pieces of what felt like a shattered life. This meant trying to begin her training in Boston and focus on her present life while still constantly caught up in the emotions and memories from the past. Removed from her home and separated from family and friends, Kayla faced what would be only one of the many difficult matches of her life:

First Practice in Boston

I didn't think it would be that hard. I thought judo would be the easiest thing for me. I thought my body wouldn't betray me, that it would stay on automatic pilot.

But of course as soon as the smell hits my nose, so do the memories. It's funny how your body instinctively reacts to certain sights, certain smells.

The smell of sweat mixed with tatami (judo mats) causes my heart to pick up speed and my body to tense. My mind replays images of my past. Practice after practice; broken bone after broken bone; fight after fight.

The tears threaten to come, and I look to Brian for support. It's been less than 30 seconds and I'm already on the verge of tears.

As soon as we come in, Jimmy greets us. He's sort of blurry to me; my eyes are swimming in wetness. He invites Mom and me into his office. Brian goes to suit up for practice.

As he begins talking all I can do is stare at his chest. His gi (judo uniform) is wide open, and I notice he's still in very good shape for a retiree. Not like Daniel, my mind quickly begins to make the comparisons. His chest is also shaved. He's staring at me with that look that I despise . . . pity.

It's written all over his face, and it only encourages my tears. I don't want his pity . . . he has no idea who I am. He wouldn't look at me if he knew the truth, if he knew what I've done.

Adjusting to a New Normal

It's quite common for victims of CSA to say that the relief they feel about their abuse having ended is overshadowed by the "new normal" they have to contend with. It is also still common to hear that the disclosure process caused a further rift between the child and parent(s), whom they see as having not protected them sufficiently from societal forces they had no way to anticipate or stand up against. Kayla, like many victims, initially saw her mother's rage at Daniel and march to the police station as being more about her own revenge and less about her daughter's well-being. Kayla felt swept up in pressures and choices she could not fully comprehend or digest and saw no way to express her own confusion about pressing charges against Daniel; she simply could not slow the process down and again felt unseen and helpless.

Victims typically describe feeling bewildered by shifts in their personal relationships and daily routines postdisclosure, along with an acute sense of being exposed. What was once private and had at times perhaps even felt special is now public and clearly wrong and can feel both shaming and stressful. For Kayla, her decision to prosecute, the need to testify, and the backdrop of the ongoing court proceedings all profoundly affected her first year in Boston, leading up to the culmination of Daniel's sentencing. She was depressed and in the middle of an emotional crisis that is not atypical once a victim of sexual abuse breaks her silence. In the next chapter, we delve more deeply into some of the longer-term psychological repercussions of disclosure, which can be quite serious and persistent in the weeks and months before and after child welfare determinations and initial court actions have been resolved.

> It's important not to assume that "the worst is over" once the legal and judicial process is either well under way or completed.

Reconciling Their Own Desire to Save Themselves with Others' Desire for Retribution

For Kayla, the judicial repercussions ended less than 6 months after she first disclosed the abuse to Brian, but she continued to experience a great deal of ambivalence and dread in general both during this period and again as the trial approached. This is not surprising when the child, who has shared an ongoing relationship with the abusive adult, feels a tremendous amount of guilt in pursuing criminal charges against the offender.

August 27, 2007 (age 17)

Dear God,

It seems like the closer I get to the trial the more I dread it. I'm so scared, God. I know exactly what's gonna happen. We're gonna get there, he's gonna walk in the door, and I'm going to freeze.

I can't do it, God. I can't betray him more than I already have. Nobody understands that he is not the one who needs punishing, I am. I did all of this, not him. Now I don't know what to do.

Love always,

Kayla

Retribution and the protection of others were not in Kayla's mind when she disclosed what was happening to her; she wasn't thinking beyond saving herself. But then others rushed to punish and blame Daniel. Because she hadn't had the opportunity to consider fully how society would respond to Daniel's actions, she was faced with again trying to reconcile the fact that someone who had violated her for 4 years was also someone she had come to depend on. Did saving herself have to mean prosecuting—and persecuting—the person she had been tied to for so long?

Having Their Day in Court

The benefits of victims having their "day in court" are widely touted, and Kayla's decision to go to trial was certainly a significant step in her personal recovery, although being better prepared for it might have made a positive difference to her recovery. While pursuing criminal charges is not necessary for recovery (and is not an option available to all victims; see the box on page 121), victims of sexual assault (whether in childhood or adulthood) generally say they find some psychological benefit in facing the person that hurt them and having the opportunity to formally break their silence about the trauma they endured.

Kayla gained strength by ultimately facing Daniel in court. By the time Daniel pleaded guilty and accepted a plea deal of 10 years of prison time, in February 2008, she had already been hospitalized psychiatrically in Boston and was barely beginning to recover from the years of pain and confusion connected to her sexual abuse. Nonetheless, facing Daniel again and talking to the judge directly was another contest in life that Kayla felt then, and feels now, that she fought and won:

February 28, 2008 (age 17)

I am awake. It is February 28, 2008. It is a Thursday. I am on my couch in my old house. I am not in my old room on my old bed. Mom sold it shortly after I moved to Boston. Probably for the best. Although I dreamed big dreams from that twin mattress, I also lived a nightmare.

It has been 288 days since I moved. It has been the worst 288 days of my life. And today will be the worst. Yesterday my mother and I went to Kohl's. I needed something to wear, you see. We leave with ugly brown pants and a green patterned top. I hate these clothes. The shirt makes me look like a turtle. I think this but do not complain. I do not fight. I am numb.

Taylor, Heather, and Kristy are all at my house. My old house. We have spent so many days here laughing, playing, gossiping, and growing. That time we put on a play of the Grinch Who Stole

WHAT ABOUT VICTIMS WHO ARE NOW ADULTS?

We see many young adults in our practices who are dealing with issues related to sexual assault that were disclosed only after they had turned 18. Their families often don't know what adversities transpired earlier in their lives, and these victims may or may not want to disclose to their families at this juncture. In light of the reality that the reporting mandate does not extend to child sexual abuse discovered or disclosed once the child has become an adult, clinicians are not required to report an allegation of child abuse unless there is a compelling reason to believe other children may be at risk of abuse by the same perpetrator (see Statutes of Limitations for Sexual Assault by Brittany Ericksen and Ilse Knech, available from *https://tinyurl.com/h5y7ftp,* for specifics on state statutes). Does this mean that criminal prosecution is off the table

Not necessarily. For victims who still want to have their day in court, most states have expanded the statute of limitations for childhood sexual abuse so that the clock does not start running for bringing criminal charges until the identity of the alleged abuser is revealed. The statute of limitation in many states used to be 10 years from the time the abuse actually occurred, regardless of when it was formally disclosed. This meant that if a child was abused at the age of 6 and only felt safe enough to file charges once he or she turned 18, the statute of limitations would have expired. In recognition of the common time lag between the occurrence of sexual assault and disclosure, many states have changed their laws so that victims have sufficient time post-disclosure to figure out what, if anything, they want to do about holding their perpetrator accountable.

Many victims are not interested in pursuing a legal option so long after their abuse occurred. Does this mean their recovery suffers from missing their day in court? Many people who choose not to prosecute as adults nonetheless feel reassured to learn that this opportunity is still available. Some choose instead to take informal actions, such as writing their perpetrators letters, arranging to confront them directly, or holding them responsible by finally telling others about this person's abusive behaviors, which may often be equally satisfying.

Therapy that child and adolescent victims receive is also available to adults. Such therapy with a trained clinician can often provide a forum for adults who disclose their sexual abuse to do the emotional processing they might not have done before and, via this process, make informed decisions about if and in what ways they want to hold the perpetrator accountable.

Christmas; the time Taylor dared me to go out on my roof in my underwear in the dead of winter; that summer where we spent every waking moment in the pool or on the deck, working on our tans; the party we had just last year, where Taylor fell in love with Teddy, Kristy fell in love with my dog, and Heather fell in love with rum.

Brian squeezes my hand and I am brought back from the past. Taylor is doing my hair. It is straightened and teased, and the room smells of hairspray. Heather and Kristy alternate putting on my makeup and drying my eyes. I have the sick thought that this could have been my wedding day.

Mimi comes over to pick up Wesley and Rose for school. They are much too young and much too fragile to be anywhere near me these days. I wonder if they know. I wonder what it's like for them to have a crazy sister. Mimi gives me a kiss and tells me she will meet us at the courthouse. Wesley and Rose hug me goodbye. I start to cry again.

We all climb in the Armada. It is the car I learned to drive in. It is the car that I will always remember. I get to ride in the front. As a child that was always my privilege as the oldest, but today I am not privileged, I am pitied. There is music on. Timbaland and One Republic are saying it's too late to apologize, it's too late, and I am wishing they would all stop singing along to it. How can they sing? On a day like this? Of course they can sing. They are still so young, and carefree. They are in a bad moment, yes, but their lives are filled with good ones, they are happy. I wish I could remember what that feels like.

The courthouse looms. There are over 20 reporters waiting like hounds as we pull in. Kristy, Heather, and Taylor form a protective circle around me as Brian practically carries me to the courthouse doors. Mom stops to say a few words of course. I feel like I am watching my life unfold but not participating . . . like this is a movie and any minute the credits will roll.

The U.S. Attorney, Laura, and the FBI agent, Patrick, are waiting in the lobby. The large building seems ancient and modern at the same time. I feel myself start to sweat through the green patterned shirt. Laura says we can go in early and look around or get comfortable if we like. I nod and Brian leads the way down the hall.

At the threshold I can see countless reporters with their pins and their recorders. My eyes sweep over my father's side of the family, all there on time waiting to watch the show. I see a bailiff. I see his lawyers. I see his parents. I panic.

I turn around and almost fall in my rush to leave. I am sobbing and can barely see as I round the corner and find a bench to collapse on. Brian is next to me and trying to soothe me. I try to control my sobs and say, " Ca . . . ca . . . call Jimmy." He dials the number. It rings. No answer. I click redial. It rings.

"Hello."

"Jimmy." I sob, "Jimmy, I can't do this. I can't do this. I can't do this."

"Kayla Kayla Kayla, slow down, take it easy, kid. Calm down. Calm down. Just breathe. Listen to my voice. Breathe."

I inhale.

"Breathe out. Breathe, kid. Listen and breathe. You are gonna go in there. You are gonna look at the judge and only the judge. And you are gonna say what you need to say. You are gonna get this shit off your chest. You are gonna be honest and just tell the truth. You are gonna get some closure so you can come back here and put this behind you, okay, kid? You hear me? Breathe."

I breathe. Laura says it's starting. I tell Jimmy I have to go. Thank you, I say. He tells me to call him after. I promise I will. "Go get 'em, kid. Be honest. Look at the judge. Breathe," he says.

My mom is on one side and Brian is on the other when I walk into the courtroom and see him for the first time. He is in a suit. His mother and father are behind him. I cry out and almost collapse, but Brian's arms stay true. I slide into the bench.

We all rise as Judge Rose comes in. I try to focus, but all I can think about is him sitting 5 feet from me. I want to scream. I want to run. I want to be anywhere but here.

Laura tells the court that my mother and the victim, K.H., will speak. My mother will go first. She gets up and walks to the stand. She pulls out her prepared speech. She talks about Daniel as a trusted family friend. She talks about how much we cared about him, how much she trusted him. She talks about all the money we spent and the travel I did because of him. She talks about her betrayal and how she thought he was her friend. She talks about how she is broken by this.

I am angry. Angry with them all, but anger can only last so long. She says thank you, Judge Rose, for allowing me to speak today, and allowing me to remind the court that a man took advantage of a young girl with a dream.

I think I will vomit.

Then the judge calls K.H. up. I sway as I make my way up to the stand. I keep my eyes on the judge. I can feel his eyes on me. They are burning into me, but I do not look. I do not falter.

"Please try and keep your voice up, young lady," the judge says. I nod and shakily begin.

"I met Daniel when I was 8 years old . . ."

By the end I am sobbing and my breathing is fast. I falter through the last bit . . . "I loved him. I think I still do . . . what was once my passion has become my prison . . . and no one will ever be able to change that. I am broken," I say.

I look up and the judge thanks me. I walk back to my seat with my eyes down.

I lean on my Mimi and cry. I hear Daniel's lawyer talking about a special bond, and I cry harder. I hear him say that he knows these two people are in love. He says he wants the court to know Daniel is sorry and so he wants Daniel to come up and say a few words if the judge will allow it.

"I stand before you today humiliated, ashamed, deeply saddened . . ." The words come out of his mouth, and I cannot stop staring. I cannot comprehend what he is saying.

"I apologize to Kayla, who I never meant to hurt . . .

"I'm deeply sorry to my parents, whose love I can never repay . . . I'm deeply sorry for the sport of judo . . . all my friends I may have lost . . . I wish I could stop this pain . . . Thank you, your honor." He sits.

Now the judge is speaking. It is time for the sentencing.

"What I do is much more than make a cold black and white calculation . . . the court has to consider many factors . . . I have heard people who respect you and value you. I have also heard people who basically, their lives, their family lives have been ruined by your actions . . . I'm not concluding that throughout your life you have been a monster . . . But when I look at your history and the nature of and circumstances of this offense the walls come tumbling down.

"You were given the opportunity, and I think you would agree the privilege of working with bright, young, talented, skilled people, people that you taught to excel . . . But it is the court's opinion that *you made a very, very serious mistake. I too hope that someday those affected can forgive you. I'm worried that this victim's life can never be repaired. She obviously cannot relive her childhood. She cannot relive those tender years. Those have been taken away from her . . ."*

Daniel stands.

"After considering all of the factors of sentencing under 18 USC 3553 and pursuant to the Sentencing Reform Act of 1984, it will be the judgment of this court that Daniel Doyle is committed to the custody of the United States Bureau of Prisons to serve the full term of 120 months."

They are putting him in cuffs. He is walking away. Right before he goes through the door he turns to me.

"I love you."

My world goes black.

Now, looking back and recalling that moment when Daniel was sentenced, Kayla writes:

It was bittersweet. It was definitely closure. I needed to get up in front of the judge and him and say my piece. I explained to the judge that what once was my passion (judo) is now my prison. It was one of the toughest days of my life. It was heart wrenching. I didn't know what to feel, and that made it worse. Everyone was so happy, so excited. Everybody had been so angry for so long. To everyone else that was the end . . . they could move on with their lives. But it wasn't that easy for me.

5

Recovery

A LONG AND WINDING ROAD

For most victims of child sexual abuse, the suffering does not end with disclosure or when a child welfare agency steps in or criminal proceedings begin. In fact, it sometimes gets worse before it gets better. Unfortunately, however, victims and those who care for them often unrealistically expect the child to be free of the pain caused by the abuse once the actual abuse ends. Youngsters we treat frequently don't even recognize that they are continuing to experience acute and prolonged distress related to their abuse, saying that they "just wanted this to be over . . . to not affect me anymore." Sometimes they also view acknowledging any ongoing distress as letting the perpetrator "win." Many youth, therefore, like Kayla, continue to at least initially suffer in silence, without access to the help they need to minimize the long-term damage of childhood abuse. They may deny the lower-level symptoms they are experiencing, only to have their distress escalate when they find they can no longer white-knuckle their way to recovery.

From all outward appearances, Kayla was competent enough to return to judo practice and the daily routines of her new life in Boston. On the inside, however, she was falling apart, the 4 years of sexual abuse continuing to take an extensive toll on her thoughts, moods, beliefs, and aspirations. While friends and family had hoped that Daniel's arrest would be a watershed in Kayla's life, she knew personally while standing in court at one of the preliminary hearings that her demons would not be swept away that easily:

126

The very first one, right before I moved to Boston—the restraining-order hearing—was the worst. Daniel came to court, and they asked me to come up and explain why I wanted a restraining order and all that. And his attorney starts cross-examining me, basically, at the restraining-order hearing, and saying, "Well, how old were you when you went on this trip?" So he was like, "So you were 16, so you were old enough to know. Would you say you were old enough to know better?" And so I was like "Uh, well . . ." I started crying. The judge had to stop him, and then she basically just said to him, "This is not about what he's being charged with; this is about staying away from her, so you have no business bringing that into the courthouse." But he was, right now, and the guy was trying to rip into me. And then the only other time I saw Daniel was at the sentencing.

Given that victims often struggle with their own confusion about why they were "chosen" by the perpetrator, about whether their victimization was their own fault, and in some cases have remained silent for a period of time about their abuse, how they are treated and responded to by parents, friends, agencies, and courts can have a critical impact on their short-term well-being and longer-term recovery.

So can many other factors. Kayla didn't want to be in Boston, living with strangers. She didn't even want to train anymore. Day and night, Kayla would think about what was happening to Daniel and how this was all *her fault*. She swung between the depths of regret and shame and bouts of relief, and these mood swings were hard for her to predict and understand and even harder to talk about. Again she took to writing about her hidden, ongoing emotional pain and conflict:

April 15, 2008 (age 17)

Dear God,

Hi. How are you, Lord? I'm all right, although I don't still know if I did that right thing or the wrong thing . . .
Did Daniel really love me?
I put him in prison; is that the right thing? How can I ever know if it was really my fault or not . . . I would appreciate your help with this . . .

Love Always,
Kayla

Withstanding sexual abuse at the hands of someone who is known and trusted leaves children confused, demoralized, and frequently unable to fully function in their daily lives. For Kayla, it took the urging and support of her ever-vigilant new coaches, family, and teammates in Boston for her to accept that she needed professional help to deal with her enduring symptoms of what was later diagnosed as PTSD and depression. Only with such help, her coaches realized, would she be freed from the tangled web of associations between her abuse at Daniel's hands and her beloved sport of judo and be able to reclaim her dreams. What to expect along the victim's path to recovery and how to recognize the signs that professional help and support from family and close friends are needed is an important issue and the topic of this chapter.

FEELING WORSE AT FIRST

As mentioned in Chapter 4, sexual abuse victims often tell us that their "new normal" after disclosure is in some ways initially worse in that they now have many more adults involved in directing their life and they have to contend with a loss of privacy and sometimes unwanted ramifications for their abuser. Prolonged abuse can create a constellation of symptoms in children, such as the following, that you may notice for the first time after disclosure, precisely because children often feel more instead of less distressed at this juncture:

- *Trouble with managing emotions.* Is your child having anger outbursts or periods of unexplained sobbing? Does she seem more irritable when things don't go as expected or defensive at the slightest perceived criticism?
- *Zoning out or being forgetful.* Does your child seem to space out in the middle of conversations or to forget things you were sure he should remember?
- *Getting down on herself.* Does your formerly self-assured child now refer to herself as "bad" or "worthless" or say no one likes her or she doesn't fit in?
- *Preoccupied with the abuser's well-being.* Does the child surprise you by defending the person who has hurt him so much? Talk about having to "make this up" to the abuser or claim that he's the guilty one?

- *Having relationship problems.* Is your child suddenly declining invitations from friends or acting reckless socially?
- *Loss of faith in the world.* Is your child or teen refusing to go to your usual house of worship or acting cynical about others or herself?

It's not surprising that repeated victimization leaves scars. What surprises many parents, law enforcement, and child welfare personnel is that the event that ends the abuse itself does not bring instant relief from the emotional damage. If you see the preceding signs from your child following disclosure, seriously consider getting professional help for the child, as discussed in Chapter 6. Meanwhile, continue to offer understanding and support.

KEEP THE OPEN DIALOGUE GOING

Even though caregivers and involved authorities alike often take actions at this time that they assume will make the victim feel better, these interventions can miss their mark because they don't fully address the depth and scope of the victim's psychological distress. Yes, the child needs your comfort and protection, but she also may, counter-intuitively, show anxiety about whether her abuser will be all right. Certainly, a child who has been abused needs to feel your understanding and empathy, but she may above all need you to *ask* how she's feeling, and *not assume* you know. An abused child might need your reassurance that you know she's telling the truth and then abruptly burst out with self-blame and guilt when you offer it. What is most helpful in this situation—even when children are believed and the adults and agencies in their environment respond with support and empathy—is to keep an open dialogue going that allows them to talk about the complexities of what they are experiencing.

> With child victims of sexual abuse, the most important response after disclosure is to allow them to talk openly about the depth and complexity of their emotional experiences. This often involves helping them find an experienced therapist or counselor whom they can speak to candidly and who can help them through the complex postdisclosure period.

RECOGNIZE THE CHILD'S NEED TO ADJUST
TO A HUGE SHIFT IN HER DAILY REALITY

We talked about the need to deal with a new normal in Chapter 4. Child and adolescent victims have already suffered once from an abuse of power and frequently misplaced trust in an adult. Therefore, even when the adults they disclose to respond in ways that make sense and may even be mandated by law, children need time to adjust to their rapidly changing reality. Before disclosure, the abuser was the central focus of the child's fears, longings, and actions. But from the minute of disclosure the abuser's place in the victim's life and their access to one another has typically changed forever. And for the victim, anything that renders her helpless and confused can stir up distressing reminders of the original victimization. In other words, even when the immediate response to a disclosure of abuse is handled as thoughtfully and compassionately as possible, many youngsters will continue to have difficulties as they begin the challenging process of coming to terms with all they have been through and what they have lost.

> Feeling helpless and confused by the new realities of postdisclosure life can elicit distressing reminders of the helplessness of being victimized.

Research has long shown that recovery can be slow and follow a winding path:

- A study of college students conducted by Sarah Ullman and her team at the University of Chicago in 2005 found that while 44.9% of child abuse victims said that disclosing was largely positive and constructive, 40.2% reported little change in how they felt in the immediate aftermath, and 15% said that disclosing made them feel worse.

- Vincent DeFrancis, in an early study of victims' reactions to disclosure done in 1969, noted that 64% of his sample expressed guilt, which was largely related to disclosure rather than the abuse experience itself.

- In their review article on CSA disclosures, Craig McNulty (1994) noted that disclosure can be related to a worsening of psychiatric symptoms under certain circumstances.

- In a 2013 study using data from a nationwide survey of childhood abuse conducted in the United Kingdom, Debra Allnock and Pam Miller found that 40% of the youthful victims they interviewed reported a "negative" disclosure experience that left them feeling more isolated and distressed in its aftermath. Most of these victims reported that their poor experiences across the "disclosure journey" were related to a lack of support and guidance from the initial people they disclosed to as well as the professionals who were later involved in their cases.

KNOW THAT TRAUMA SYMPTOMS MAY BE SIMMERING UNDER THE SURFACE

As the research evidence shows, not all abused children feel traumatized by the disclosure process. But that doesn't mean they aren't still struggling emotionally. *After disclosure, many children struggle with PTSD and other trauma-related symptoms that often, along with the abuse itself, have remained underground for a significant period of time.* Kayla remembers that it took months once she was in Boston for her to stop crying and to recapture her determination to sort through the myriad complicated emotional reactions from the abuse itself without resorting to self-destructive thoughts and behaviors. Particularly when there have been multiple incidents of abuse by a trusted adult, victims tend to develop a host of trauma-related beliefs and feelings that are difficult to shake, such as those described previously, on pages 128 and 129.

Kayla's journals from the time immediately before her revelation show that her psychological distress was escalating, but of course it was kept hidden from others around her. This can make it difficult for parents and other adults to perceive the depth of the distress that may emerge after disclosure, which is why they need to anticipate it. As the journal entries immediately following her 16th birthday reveal, Kayla's thoughts of suicide and feelings of depression had become a mainstay of her existence, leading up to her disclosing the abuse later that year:

July 6, 2006 (age 16)

Dear God,

Hi. It's me. How are you? As of right now I'm all right. I'm on my way to San Jose, California, for the Junior Olympics. I'm 70 kg, now my weight is good.

Well, I just finished reading all of my old entries, and it seems that not a lot has changed. I'm still depressed if not more than ever. I still think about killing myself and have almost acted on it several times. I cut myself. It wasn't for the first time and it probably won't be the last.

I wonder if other people feel like this. Like an overwhelming sadness that runs deep in their hearts, like no matter what you do it will always be there.

I have felt suicidal for little over a year now and I wonder if I started acting on it now where will I be in another year's time? Unable to write you? How long must this go on?

I'm tired of pretending like I'm happy. There're many people I love and who I know love me.

God, for some reason it feels like the love will never be able to touch the sadness inside of me. And it scares me.

Am I supposed to live life feeling this way because, if I am, I can't. Please help me conquer my demons. They wake me in the night and haunt me in the day. Please.

Love Always,
Kayla

PAY ATTENTION WHEN SYMPTOMS DO SHOW THROUGH THE VENEER

It's wise to gently ask your teen about how she is feeling even if she is keeping the symptoms of PTSD beneath the surface. This is when the open dialogue becomes so vital. This does not mean nagging your child or insisting she is distressed when, in fact, a proportion of children do report feeling better almost immediately following the revelation of their abuse. The guideline is to remain interested and curious about how the child is responding and let her know you understand and expect that she may be continuing to struggle in the aftermath of breaking her silence. You can also offer to take the teen to talk to a professional in the field if the teen is unwilling to talk with you at all; remember that we as professionals can probe in a way that parents cannot based on our

> Be open and curious rather than making assumptions about how your child is feeling, but observe closely.

cumulative experience. So, for example, in our practices we often talk with teens about the "typical" reactions we see from others in their situation, allowing them to feel less isolated and alone in their own responses.

What we hear most frequently from the abused youngsters we work with is that they feel distressed, confused, and desperate for relief both before and after their silence is broken. Kayla's description of her nightmares, suicidal thoughts, and self-loathing highlights how these symptoms went largely unreported and unrecognized, *which meant they could not be addressed*:

> *To this day I still have this nightmare: I am in Boston. My mind flashes from the past to the future very fast. I usually have a glimpse of me in the courtroom and them putting Daniel in cuffs. Him telling me he loves me. That one of us won't make it out of this alive. Then I can see the roof of my apartment. Daniel is looking in on me and I'm asleep. I can see him and I know I am sleeping but I can't move. He comes inside. He is older. He is angry. He is on top of me. I am trying to scream, but nothing will come out. He is choking me. I am dying and I can't fight back. He is choking me and saying he loves me. Usually here I wake up crying or screaming. It takes me a few moments to get oriented and realize it was just a dream.*

It's important to know that many survivors will go to the same lengths after revealing abuse as before to look and feel like they have survived the trauma and are doing well. These survivors, like Kayla, are skeptical that others will fully understand what they have been through, and their inclination is to avoid and deny the ongoing impact of the abusive relationship on their lives. Kayla desperately did not want what had happened with Daniel to plague her going forward. As we explain later when we discuss complex PTSD, her symptoms functioned to help her avoid fully facing and accepting the impact of her past reality. This tension between wanting others to understand their ongoing distress and wanting the past to "just be over" makes it challenging for the adults in the child's life to know how and when to respond to symptoms that they observe. Triggered trauma memories and flashbacks are common for abuse victims, but often those closest to the victim have no idea what she is experiencing, as Kayla describes:

Anything can become a trigger. One time I went into a panic attack because someone on the team was wearing the same cologne that Daniel used to wear. I remember the scent hitting my nose and then it was as if there was a flood in my mind. Daniel's face, happy, screaming, smiling, lustful. I remember I broke out in a sweat and wondered if everyone could tell I was crazy. I remember the rest of that day all I could do was focus on not losing it. On just surviving and being normal until I could get home that night and cry in the shower.

Sometimes at practice I would hear his voice. I would hear him yelling at me. Telling me I was never going to make it without him. I hear him saying I can do better. That I'm not trying hard enough. I can see his face and feel his emotions.

Right before I was admitted to McLean I had a serious episode where I thought I was still in Ohio. I called Brian Daniel and kept laughing and joking with him. I don't remember any of the episode, except when I came to I was out sitting on the sidewalk in front of the judo house. Brian was terrified and called my mom. The next day she flew out and admitted me to McLean.

COULD YOUR CHILD HAVE PTSD?

Again, hidden symptoms are hard to treat. But does your child need to qualify for a psychiatric diagnosis to get the treatment she needs? This is a complicated issue. In general, the reason for standardized criteria by which psychiatrists, psychologists, and mental health clinicians can render a particular diagnosis is to ensure that the person receives the treatment that research has shown to be most effective for that disorder. But what happens if an individual has many of the symptoms of PTSD, a common consequence of child sexual abuse, but not all of the criteria required by the American Psychiatric Association's *Diagnostic and Statistical Manual of Mental Disorders*? At this point important decisions must be made about whether to take a "wait and see" approach (perhaps the symptoms will disappear or they'll increase to the point of fulfilling the formal diagnostic criteria) or treat the symptoms now to reduce the harm to the patient.

A significant proportion of youth subjected to sexual abuse will in fact develop symptoms of PTSD, which can significantly interfere with the child's emotional, mental, and behavioral stability. So of course if your child displayed them you would want to be sure they were treated effectively. The problem is that many people who have PTSD symptoms *don't* meet the criteria for a formal psychiatric diagnosis—*one* intrusive symptom related to the trauma, *one* symptom of avoidance related to the trauma, *two* symptoms of negative changes in thoughts and mood since the trauma, and *two* symptoms of hyperarousal related to the trauma. Without meeting all these criteria, a child could not be given the PTSD diagnosis, and some mental health professionals would therefore hesitate to offer targeted PTSD treatment. However, the evidence-based treatments for PTSD almost all begin with skills training for symptom management, and there's no reason children cannot receive help with symptoms like nightmares, unjustified feelings of guilt, and harmful avoidance, even if they don't have a formal PTSD diagnosis. While the child is receiving this skills training (see Chapter 6 for details), the clinician can evaluate whether it makes sense to start a second phase of treatment that typically includes exposure to remembered aspects of the trauma (also explained in Chapter 6) and is focused on reconstructing and processing details of the past sexual abuse.

Also be aware that symptoms stemming from sexual abuse trauma typically evolve over a period of time, and sometimes a child who would not qualify for a diagnosis of PTSD during abuse or immediately after it ends will meet the criteria later. According to the American Psychiatric Association, a majority of individuals exposed to a traumatic life event will experience significant short-term distress, and for sexual abuse victims, particularly when their abuse is ongoing, the chances of eventually developing PTSD are quite high—remember here that PTSD symptoms need to persist for more than a month before this diagnosis can be made. We see many youngsters in our clinical practices who believe the world is not a safe place and that they don't personally deserve a good life. When we investigate, we find that many of these beliefs can be traced back to sexual abuse by a trusted adult. But this effect often takes time to develop. The younger the child is when the abuse happens, the less likely it is that the child will fully understand that the touching that has been going on for some time is inappropriate. For many victims, like Kayla, it only dawns on them gradually. This full realization in adolescence often leads to increasing distress, which fortunately can lead to disclosure but, unfortunately, also to an increase in PTSD symptoms.

Kayla captures this evolution of her awareness about the relationship with Daniel in some of her original journal entries (see Chapters

1 and 2). Becoming fully aware of his betrayal, while also feeling confused and guilty because she still believed she had colluded in the abuse, caused her to continue to have intrusive memories, nightmares, and scary, dangerous dissociative episodes long past the point that others expected that she would "be fine"—and the same can be true for other abused children. Although the disconnected experience of dissociation "helps" the victim block out extremely painful memories, it can also lead to an inability to experience essential emotions and remember key moments. Dissociation can also lead victims into repeated abusive relationships. For Kayla this ongoing deterioration is captured in multiple recollections of the period after her arrival in Boston and before Daniel is sentenced months later:

> Over the first weeks in Boston I was a wreck in the dojo, a puddle of tears. Judo felt dirty now, and everyone, I was sure, was staring and whispering about me. Every time I stepped on the mat, Daniel rematerialized—"What are you doing, girl? You know you can't do this without me!"—leaving me both loathing him and thinking again that I loved him—trembling over everyone's expectation that I would testify against him and lock him away.
>
> I felt as if I was going crazy. Panic frequently seized my chest and closed around my windpipe. Anything could trigger it: the smell of Daniel's cologne on a stranger, a song we used to listen to, a screaming coach.
>
> One night I jumped in my car to escape before something terrible happened, afraid even to stop for gas because the people at the station would know my secret, then drove south on the interstate to start a new life until I finally pulled over, even more scared of what I would do without judo.
>
> Another night, in a blizzard, a panic attack sent me crawling out my window onto the garage roof and leaping down to the yard to evade my worried teammates downstairs, then scrambling through the neighborhood and into a nearby nature reserve.
>
> I later learned that Brian, terrified that I had taken an overdose of sleeping pills, bashed down my locked bedroom door, and then, seeing I was gone, he and seven teammates jumped into three cars to pursue me, a police car joining the hunt.

Kayla's journal from this time emphasizes how complex the emotional aftermath of a disclosure can be. Kayla continued to feel ambivalent about the disclosure and its repercussions for Daniel and to feel attached to him, which led her to seek contact with him after arriving in Boston. No one in her immediate network of friends and family had any idea, and they undoubtedly would have been both shocked and disapproving. Kayla's running off and being chased by her friends and the police, it turned out, followed Brian's discovery that she had been secretly talking to Daniel via a burner phone that she had purchased:

June 18, 2007

Dear God,

Well, a lot has happened. I'm going to come clean about the big stuff.

When Brian was in Italy I talked to him [Daniel]. I called him and he answered. I hung up. I called him again and he answered. This time he knew it was me.

We talked. We talked about everything. I was so lonely and I need him so much. I missed him. Daniel has always been the rock in my life. He always will be.

So he told me to go buy a phone and use fake stuff and cash, so I did. And then I called him the next night. And the night after that. And the next one. We talked for hours just like we used to, and it made me remember the good times.

But this time something was different. I needed him a little less and he needed me a little more. Lord, please forgive me, because I lied. I told him I wouldn't testify. I don't want to, but I know they will make me. I told him I still love him.

It's like when you cut off your leg—but sometimes still think it's there. I called him tonight and I could tell he was drunk from the smell of his breath over the phone. Please help me need him less.

Love Always,
Kayla

Kayla was noticing that the focus of her life was changing. Her friends and family thought it had already shifted 180 degrees, and they might have been able to help her (or find a professional who could help her) deal with her confusing emotions if they had understood that the shift can take time, especially when the abuse went on for as long as it had. More knowledge about the aftermath of disclosure might have allowed a caring adult to convey to her that ambivalence is understandable; that understanding, in turn, might have relieved her distress and confusion enough to avoid triggering some of her more potentially self-destructive behaviors like climbing out a window in the dark. While the more adults know, the more effective they can be in listening to and supporting a child who has suffered and disclosed sexual victimization, even this awareness does not guarantee that victims, like Kayla, will not require professional help to lessen their distress and the problem behaviors they may be using to cope with that distress. As Kayla's mother says:

> "After your abuse was disclosed, I worried about you more. I was concerned for your psychological well-being because we felt like you had been, in a sense, brainwashed by Daniel. I was worried because you would call home and tell us you weren't good enough anymore. Also some of your friends in Boston were concerned that you were continuing to talk with Daniel even though you told us you weren't. After much nagging on my part, you finally broke down and admitted you had the burner phone, and I believe it was then I came back to Boston to get you into treatment."

Common Short-Term Symptoms to Watch For

As noted earlier, distress needs to be addressed whether or not the individual has been given a PTSD diagnosis. Consider nightmares. Although nightmares about the abuse alone would not qualify a victim for a PTSD diagnosis, it is clear to parents, teachers, and those of us in the mental health area who work with children on a daily basis that a child with chronic nightmares and disrupted sleep is *not* a child who can function effectively and feel happy and successful in his daily life. The same is true for a victim who continues to seek contact with her abuser.

> When a child has been traumatized, the specific diagnosis is less important than perceiving the level of individual distress and how we can help the child with it.

As noted earlier, most victims of repeated sexual abuse have some symptoms of an acute stress response and/or PTSD symptoms both *during* and *in the period following the revelation of* their abuse. Everyone in their immediate network needs to remain vigilant when a child or teen who has been sexually traumatized is experiencing *any* of the following symptoms or, more important, evidences specific changes in behavior that cause the victim at least moderate distress. Behavioral changes to be aware of following the initial disclosure period (see the box below), particularly if these persist for longer than 1 month, are:

- The development of new fears
- Separation anxiety, particularly in young children
- Sleep disturbance or nightmares
- Unexplained sadness
- Loss of interest in normal activities
- Reduced concentration, especially for typically enjoyed activities
- A decline in schoolwork
- Unexplained anger
- New medical complaints with no clear physical cause
- Unexplained, new irritability

Many of the short-term responses to trauma are predictable and not necessarily serious, such as temporarily sleeping poorly or having trouble concentrating, and may disappear eventually without formal treatment. But the only way to ensure that they don't worsen and interfere with the youth's healing is to monitor these problems. Children who have suffered the horror of repeated sexual abuse, particularly by someone in a position of authority and trust, are less likely to recover quickly, and reclaim their earlier level of functioning, than those who have had other traumatic experiences. *This is why ongoing attention is so crucial. Recovery is not achieved when the abuse ends; it is just beginning.*

THE TIME FRAME FOR SYMPTOMS OF DISTRESS

When mental health practitioners try to determine whether a child should be diagnosed with PTSD, the time factor is important yet tricky to consider. With sexual abuse, it is not apparent when the trauma actually begins or ends. But having symptoms like those listed above for up to a month is usually viewed as what is called an acute stress response. If the symptoms develop and persist for a longer time, the practitioner will consider a diagnosis of PTSD.

Longer-Term Harms of Child Sexual Abuse

Victims like Kayla are likely to have nightmares, become extremely fearful, and have other behavioral symptoms like those listed previously, and the earlier they receive appropriate treatment for them—with or without a diagnosis of PTSD—the more quickly they can be resolved. Chapter 6 explains what types of treatment can help and how to get an expert evaluation and diagnosis.

Unfortunately, child sexual abuse is also often associated with a range of other difficulties later in life, including low self-esteem, severe anxiety, phobias, eating disorders, self-destructive behaviors, substance use, and a variety of physical disorders. Whether resolving the short-term behavioral symptoms right away can prevent these long-term outcomes from developing is not entirely clear. It appears that the longer the abuse continues, the more severe it is, the closer to the child the perpetrator was, and the more helplessly trapped the child felt during the abuse, the more likely the trauma is to have long-lasting effects. Fortunately, the effective treatments we have today make recovery possible for the great majority of children. But we reiterate that it is so important to notice problematic symptoms early and address them promptly and persistently.

Here are some highlights of recent research on the longer-term effects of child sexual abuse:

- Individuals who were sexually abused as children have been found to be three to four times more likely to report lifetime problems with major depression when compared to individuals without histories of childhood abuse, according to Frank Putnam and a host of other researchers, as reported in 2003.

- Child sexual abuse that was reported after the abuse had ended was associated with higher levels of adult depression, anxiety, and ongoing PTSD symptoms across all age groups studied by Beth Molnar and her colleagues, using the National Comorbidity Survey data, in 2001.

- Psychiatric disorders were nearly 50% more common among the women in Molnar's study who reported a history of childhood abuse than in those with no childhood abuse history.

- Sexual victimization in childhood or adolescence increases the likelihood of sexual victimization in adulthood between 2 and 13.7 times, according to reliable studies, including those conducted by psychologists Kevin Lalor and Rosaleen McElvaney in 2010 at the Dublin Institute of Technology.

Complex PTSD

Years of doctors' observations and research studies have shown that childhood sexual abuse has predictable short-term effects and common long-term effects. But it also gradually became clear that severe, sustained abuse caused damage beyond the symptoms of PTSD as defined by the *DSM*. From this realization emerged the term *complex posttraumatic stress disorder* (C-PTSD) to describe a constellation of more far-reaching and multifaceted symptoms. This term was first used in the psychiatric literature in 1992 by Judith Herman 12 years after PTSD first became a formal, recognized diagnosis, and although it's still not recognized as a formal diagnosis in the *DSM-5*, this syndrome has been well researched as an important entity in carefully conducted clinical research, as supported by Bessel van der Kolk and colleagues in a comprehensive 2009 review of this literature.

Specifically, complex PTSD results from exposure to repeated, severe, and chronic trauma(s) from which it is difficult for the victim to escape—as is frequently true for sexual abuse that occurs in childhood (as opposed to adulthood, where trauma more often involves a single incident with a stranger or is reported sooner to authorities). Its symptoms fall into seven domains identified in a 2005 review by Dr. Alexandra Cook and colleagues at the Justice Resource Institute (based on a 2003 white paper from the National Child Traumatic Stress Network Complex Trauma Task Force):

- *Attachment*—problems with relationship boundaries, lack of trust, social isolation, difficulty perceiving and responding to other's emotional states, and lack of empathy.
- *Biology*—sensory-motor developmental dysfunction, sensory-integration difficulties, somatization, and increased medical problems.
- *Affect or emotional regulation*—poor affect regulation, difficulty in identifying and expressing emotions and internal states, and difficulties in communicating needs, wants, and wishes.
- *Dissociation*—amnesia, depersonalization, discrete states of consciousness with discrete memories, affect, and functioning, and impaired memory for state-based events.

- *Behavioral control*—problems with impulse control, aggression, pathological self-soothing, and sleep problems.

- *Cognition*—difficulty regulating attention, problems with a variety of "executive functions," such as planning, judgment, initiation, use of materials, and self-monitoring, difficulty processing new information, difficulty focusing and completing tasks, poor object constancy, problems with "cause–effect" thinking, and language developmental problems, such as a gap between receptive and expressive communication abilities.

- *Self-concept*—fragmented and disconnected autobiographical narrative, disturbed body image, low self-esteem, excessive shame, and negative internal working models of self.

Although these terms are somewhat abstract, they give you an idea of how far-reaching the effects of sexual abuse can be in the most severe cases. The abused child or teen may have trouble forming or keeping the normal relationships she had before the abuse started. She may have nightmares and insomnia, gaps in memory, or feel disconnected from reality. She might be impulsive or aggressive, emotionally volatile, and have trouble concentrating and learning. Medical problems and illnesses might crop up without any traceable physical cause. Feeling down on themselves, easily ashamed, and negative is common among long-term abuse victims. As dire as this may sound, *good treatment is available, and the sooner symptoms are addressed, the more quickly they can be resolved and the child or teen can recover.*

NO LONGER ALONE: INCHING TOWARD PROFESSIONAL HELP

Kayla experienced many symptoms of complex PTSD, including behavioral impulsivity involving self-harm, disturbances in body image, and periods of dissociation, both before and after her disclosure. These symptoms came to the attention of Kayla's coaches in Boston shortly after her arrival. In thinking back about the first weeks that Kayla lived and trained with them in Boston, the Pedros, both father and son, recall how troubled she appeared to be and remember clearly their mounting worry that, without professional help, Kayla would neither be safe nor able compete at the level she aspired to:

"Kayla wanted to quit judo, to disengage from every part of her life," recalls Jimmy Pedro Junior, who said he remembers receiving a panicked call one night not long after Kayla arrived in Boston after she had climbed up onto a roof and was threatening to jump; another time, Pedro Junior recalls, she ran away and could not be found for quite some time."

These behaviors scared both Kayla's coaches and her teammates, and they began talking with her about seeking professional help, a suggestion that Kayla initially rejected. But the Pedros persevered and, refusing to be daunted by Kayla's protests, moved forward with a plan to make sure she accepted the help she needed, even making this a requirement for continued judo training:

"She was in a bad place when she showed up," Pedro Junior said of Kayla. "Her whole world was upside down, and I think she wanted to just sort of disappear. But that girl is a fighter. We eventually got her enrolled in high school. My father and I took on the role of pseudo-parents. We got her talking to a therapist who was also one of our judo students, Dr. Blaise Aguirre, who is also world-renowned for his work with abuse victims, and slowly, she started to come around."

It was fortunate for Kayla that the adults in her life at that point did not grant her more time to struggle alone with her distress. Studies have shown that PTSD can resolve gradually or spontaneously without specialized treatment, but complex PTSD generally does not, especially when it includes symptoms of self-harm and suicidal thinking. At that time Kayla was experiencing periods of dissociation, self-harming behaviors, suicidal thinking, and a deep sense of despair and self-loathing—all characteristic of complex PTSD. In fact Kayla's symptoms had become so severe in the aftermath of her disclosure that, without professional intervention, her condition would likely have deteriorated further.

> It often takes a worsening of symptoms, along with the resolve of concerned adults, for child victims to finally accept that they will need expert help to recover fully and thrive.

Luckily for Kayla, the Pedros were principled in all the ways Daniel had been disreputable. They set appropriate boundaries and helped Kayla mend, insisting, together with Kayla's mother, that she agree to an admission at McLean Hospital so as to receive the top-notch psychiatric care she needed. But it was still no easy task for Kayla to agree to even a brief stay at McLean, as she worried that taking time out for treatment was an admission of weakness and would also derail her training and dreams of becoming an Olympian. Fortunately for Kayla, she and the Pedros already knew and trusted one of us, Dr. Aguirre, a psychiatrist who is the medical director of a program at McLean designed to help young adults like Kayla recover from trauma-related problems.

The long-standing relationship with the Pedros, along with the availability of a specialized treatment option at McLean Hospital just miles from where Kayla lived and trained, made obtaining professional help possible. In fact to this day I (Blaise Aguirre) feel fortunate that my relationship with the Pedros and love for judo made it possible for me to first meet and then help Kayla get the intensive help she needed shortly after arriving in Boston. As I recall,

> "In 2007, Olympic judo bronze medalist Jimmy Pedro came to me with a very specific and confidential request, but in order to get to that here is the context.
>
> "I have always loved the sport of judo and as a medical student in South Africa had practiced it regularly. I also believed in its philosophy. The word *judo* itself means the gentle way, and is in a sense a contradiction: Judo is the art of nonresistance in the face of aggression. The idea is that, when attacked, you take the anger and action of the other to use against him. The idea of gentle yet effective combat resonated with my perspectives on therapy and my appreciation and application of the treatment I use, one known as dialectical behavior therapy or DBT, a therapy that integrates the Eastern acceptance principles of Zen with the Western therapy of behaviorism.
>
> "Some years after I arrived in the United States I read that Jimmy had won an Olympic medal and was teaching at a gym just up the road from me in Wakefield, Massachusetts. I trained with him from 1998 to 2008 before the demands of my psychiatry practice and ageing body got the better of regular attendance. Nevertheless I had grown close to Jimmy and his family. However, it was that day in 2007 that stands out in my mind. 'We have a kid coming to train with us. She is great, but she was

abused by her coach. She is very emotional and has a hard time being on the mat. Her mother is very worried about her and so are we. Can you help?'

"I met Kayla at the gym. She was serious and dedicated. She trained unlike any other judo player. Each movement precise, each with the same accurate technique, repetition after repetition, rarely resting, never talking or goofing off like the rest of us. She acknowledged that she had been struggling with nightmares, flashbacks, difficult intrusive memories, long crying spells, difficulty sleeping, loss of appetite, and despair. She was someone who had PTSD and perhaps an episode of major depression. I understood the concern of Jimmy and Kayla's mother, and I had the further worry that she might become so despondent and hopeless that she could end up carrying through with her incessant thoughts of self-destructiveness if she did not get professional help.

"With that concern in mind, I referred Kayla to our adolescent residential unit. She needed to rest and get professional help. Because she was so diligent in her learning of judo, I had no doubt that she would similarly learn some of the techniques that we taught our patients to deal with symptoms similar to hers."

Taking a Break in Pursuit of Recovery

What Kayla and other sexual abuse victims need help in recognizing and accepting is that *someone victimized in childhood must, at times, stop his or her daily routine in order to focus fully on treatment and recovery.* Without this pause, victims often remain stuck in cycles where their considerable and unresolved distress leads to escalating avoidance, dissociation, and an undue reliance on destructive coping strategies. The decision to seek professional help was extremely grueling for Kayla even with the unified support of her coaches and family, as she continued not only to question whether she needed therapy in the first place but also to feel deeply ashamed and fearful of placing her faith in yet another new group of people.

Looking back, Kayla remembers only too well the arm-twisting from her mother, who flew to Boston at the last minute to ensure that she accepted the residential admission she now so desperately needed. And Kayla also recalls well the anger she felt toward the very same people who were trying to help her, including the last-ditch efforts to reverse her mother's decision about the admission, a decision Kayla now feels may well have saved her life:

> Even though I agreed to be evaluated, I freaked out once I realized what was really happening, sobbing and screaming as my mother turned her back and left me on the ward. "I will go back to judo," I remember pleading, "I will do <u>anything</u>; please just don't leave me here."
>
> And then she was gone and there was nowhere left to run . . . I was once again alone, alone and frightened and exhausted from the battle I had been waging for such a long time.
>
> That night I remember reluctantly talking to my therapist, Jen, and realizing that she was there to just listen and that the other girls on the unit had even worse problems than me.
>
> And I began thinking that maybe, just maybe, this could help.

Understanding the available options and approaches to the treatment of PTSD and complex PTSD is necessary to get the best possible help for victims of abuse, so we strongly encourage you to read the next chapter. But be aware that the initial challenge is often to help the youth (in addition to those around her, including parents) accept that the impact of childhood trauma does not end with the revelation or discovery of the abuse and that professional help can be enormously beneficial. Only with a great deal of external encouragement will many survivors acknowledge their continued suffering and accept a professional referral they may urgently need.

For many victims, the overwhelming loss of the cloak of anonymity, along with the shame and guilt that can soar to the surface of the child's emotions, often triggers self-injury and drastically lowers self-esteem. The appearance of these symptoms often brings the child's distress to our attention—and possibly to yours. For Kayla these symptoms were exacerbated by the changes in her living arrangements and relationships postdisclosure. She had struggled with suicidal thinking and extreme emotional distress for years before her revelations about Daniel, but that distress spilled over into heightened impulsivity, self-harm, and an uptick in suicidal thinking after she arrived in Boston. This is an important lesson for the adults in a victim's world that we cannot state often enough: *Disclosure may not be a relief to the child or teen.*

It may open the floodgates and impose a new normal that is extremely difficult to manage. The next lesson is just as important: Kayla eventually acquiesced to an evaluation at one of the McLean Hospital programs, but only once it became clear that her coaches and mother were not going to back away from her need for professional help.

The obvious next question is: What is the best type of professional help, and how can you find it? What we know to date is the subject of the next chapter.

6

Finding the Way
to Professional Help

July 2007 (age 17)

Dear God,

Well, a lot has happened in a month. Let's go in chronological order.

Shortly after I wrote the entry about using a burner phone to contact Daniel, Brian read it. He called my mother, who immediately took action. She flew to Boston and placed me in McLean Hospital.

To say the least I was pissed. I have no problem talking to someone but to just throw me into an institution without trying anything else? I was furious.

But I was really only going to be there for a short while, and so I did with it what I could. Upon arrival at McLean everyone has to write a symptom history. A story of your life so to speak. And for the first time in my life I was honest. I laid it all on that paper, and it just poured out of me. It felt really good.

So I'm trying to be honest now in all that I do.

So at McLean I meet Jen, who is my case manager and is going to be my therapist. I don't know how I feel about her yet. Only time will tell.

Love Always,
Kayla

For survivors of child sexual abuse, like Kayla, recognizing the need for professional help can be critical to achieving a full recovery. Knowing when to treat and what type of treatment to pursue, however, can be one of the greatest challenges that these children and their families contend with. In this chapter we explain how to get a professional evaluation for diagnosis and treatment and describe the types of treatment considered most effective for PTSD and other trauma-related symptoms. (You'll find sources of help in the Resources section.)

Kayla's experience offers a window into the treatment path that is often effective for victims of prolonged sexual abuse. Her treatment involved a 2-week admission to one of McLean Hospital's short-term adolescent residential treatment programs in which an integrated cognitive behavioral therapy (CBT) and dialectical behavioral therapy (DBT) approach is used. This combination of treatments helps patients first identify and then modify the potentially life-threatening symptoms and behaviors that they are struggling with and that plague many of them. The same treatments also help teens address non-life-threatening behaviors that are affecting their ability to function effectively in daily life, from anxiety to eating disorders and substance use.

WHEN TO SEEK PROFESSIONAL HELP

As we've discussed, the exact time at which to seek professional help is difficult to pinpoint. What we know is that children are likely to have an acute stress response following episodes of abuse, and when the abuse has been prolonged, many will develop PTSD. The trouble is that outward appearances—and outsiders' expectations—don't always reflect inner realities. You may have seen little indication of the psychological effects on your child while the abuse was taking place, and with discovery, just when you thought your child's burden would be lightened, the child's emotional distress may have gotten worse. Kayla describes the severe distress she was experiencing right before being admitted to McLean Hospital:

In the days prior to being hospitalized I was definitely at rock bottom. I had been in Boston for about 2 months and things were not going well. I was suffering severely from PTSD. Having flashbacks and nightmares. Disassociating on the mat at practice. I was *struggling with small menial tasks like waking up in the morning and brushing my teeth. Getting out of bed. I was severely depressed and felt very alone. Jimmy was concerned, as were Big Jim and Brian.*

One day I had a panic attack or a kind of flashback and I called Brian Daniel repeatedly. Brian was so worried he called my mom, and the next day she flew up to Boston and admitted me to McLean. I was horrified and scared. I had to sleep there every night, but I got to go to judo for evening sessions. There was a training camp going on and there were athletes from all over the country there. I remember feeling paranoid because they all must have known why I wasn't at the morning sessions. Brian told me to relax, that everyone just thought I was working, but I could see it in their eyes. They were all freaked out. On the second night once my mom had gone home again and before Brian drove me back to the hospital, I took Jimmy in the office and I begged him not to make me go back. I was sobbing hysterically and couldn't really even get the words out. I just didn't want to go back. I didn't want to be crazy. I didn't want to be in that place and think about everything that was wrong with my life, I wanted to forget it had ever happened. But Jimmy said no—Kayla, you need help, and the sooner you accept it and work on getting better, the sooner you can get out of there. And that's really when my mentality about McLean changed. I treated it like I treat anything in my life— like a fight. A fight I needed to win. But this time it was Me vs. Me.

In Chapter 4, we offered a brief list of internal distress signals to be alert for postdisclosure so that the child's pain does not remain secret, where it could fester, as Kayla's did. You've now also read about the constellation of symptoms that constitute the diagnoses of PTSD and complex PTSD, the latter often seen in children who have been abused for a very long time where the abuse is perpetrated by someone in a position of authority over the child. Thus, if any of these signs of distress persist for more than a month, we strongly suggest seeking professional help for the child or teen if you haven't already done so.

> Signs of internal distress that last for a month or more call for consulting a mental health professional.

If you have any doubts about whether professional help is needed, the following descriptions of the physical, emotional, and mental problems associated with complex PTSD that you read about in

Chapter 5 are repeated here in more tangible terms that you can apply to monitoring a child who has disclosed abuse. The more you can tell a mental health professional about the behaviors and emotions your child is experiencing, the more accurate the professional's assessment will be and the more appropriate the treatment prescribed.

• *Difficulties with regulating all emotions:* Includes the emotions of sadness, anger, guilt, and shame, along with related suicidal thoughts.

Does your child seem more volatile than you think was normal for her before the period when the sexual abuse occurred? Do things that would not have bothered her in the past cause a blowup? Does she clam up when you least expect silence?

• *Disruptions in the experience of awareness:* Includes forgetting and/or reliving traumatic events or problems with dissociation, including episodes of detachment and/or depersonalization.

Children who have suffered long-term abuse may be left with memory gaps about the events that took place during the time the abuse occurred that may or may not have been part of the abuse. Victims also report having the feeling that they're observing themselves from outside their body as in a movie or that things around them aren't real, or both. You may find yourself surprised when you're reliving a family incident—like a holiday gathering or something a family member did—and your "Remember when . . . ?" query is met with silence by your child. You may find it disturbing when your child seems to be distant or pauses before responding in a conversation.

• *Disruptions in self-perception:* May include the sense of being completely different from other people and/or being ineffective in daily life.

Suffering sexual abuse in childhood can leave a child feeling as if this experience sets him apart from all of his nonabused peers. It can leave a child with the sense of being "dirty" or "damaged" and incapable of being successful. Trauma-related feelings of guilt, shame, and anger can color the child's view of himself.

• *Distorted perceptions of the perpetrator:* Includes becoming preoccupied with the fate of the perpetrator and can involve being engrossed with feelings of guilt or revenge.

As is revealed so clearly in Kayla's writings, the relationship between a victim and perpetrator can be complicated and bewildering to parents and other caring adults in the child's life. Victims often feel a mixture of polarized and intense feelings for the person who abused them, and this swirl of feelings toward the perpetrator can persist for quite a long time after the abuse has stopped and been revealed.

• *Disrupted relations with others:* May include isolation, distrust, or a repeated search for a rescuer.

An abused child's view of the world as a safe and predictable place has likely been altered, which can result in a reluctance to "try again" to form intimate connections. Since the relationship with the perpetrator has often been dominant, at times a child may display a general wariness or, alternatively, what can look like recklessness in how he or she relates to others.

• *Disrupted system of meanings:* May include a disruption in faith in core beliefs about oneself and the surrounding environment.

If your child or teen does see a mental health professional to be evaluated for trauma specifically stemming from sexual abuse, what can you expect?

SAFETY FIRST

As explained in Chapter 5, many sexual abuse survivors resort to self-injury and suicidal thinking and other high-risk and impulsive behaviors as ways of managing the distressing emotions and beliefs that typically result from years of sexual victimization. Kayla started cutting herself when she was 16. After disclosing her abuse, she continued to struggle with urges to engage in self-destructive behaviors:

Right after disclosure I thought about cutting. And I thought about suicide. But mostly I was numb. I was numb to pain, the world, judo, everything. It was as if I was in a fog and nothing could pull me out. Not even the pain of cutting.

Unfortunately, even when it increases following disclosure as it often does, this heightened internal distress frequently remains hidden from others:

One way that I hid cutting from my mom was by wearing baggy clothes. I already lived in sweatpants by this point, so it was no surprise that I was wearing sweaters in the summer. I usually just cut my upper arms, my wrists, sometimes the insides of my thighs. No one ever got close enough to see the marks. And if they did, no one ever said anything. I made sure not to cut too deep. I only have one scar that's still visible on my left wrist, and every day it's a reminder to me that you can't ease pain with more pain.

Because evidence of self-injury may have remained undercover for a while, it's important for parents and others involved in a victim's life to respond quickly to any signs of self-destructive behavior or urges. It's also why the first priority for any treatment for the traumatic effects of sexual abuse will be to keep the child safe.

Understanding Cutting and Other Forms of Self-Injury

The behavior often known colloquially as "cutting" is one example of a behavior known in the field of psychology as *nonsuicidal self-injury (NSSI)*. NSSI is common among sexually abused children and teens, as well as among those who are not abused (see the box below). NSSIs are intentional acts that directly damage the body but occur without an intention to commit suicide. Although the most common form of NSSI seen in clinical practice is self-cutting, other forms of NSSI include burning, scratching, hitting, intentionally preventing wounds from healing, head banging, inserting foreign objects under the skin, and swallowing sharp objects (see the box on page 154).

NSSI: A BIG PROBLEM FOR CHILD SEXUAL ABUSE VICTIMS AND OTHERS

NSSI is not limited to those who have suffered child sexual abuse, and it is all too common, even in young children. For instance, nearly 8% of third-graders reported injuring themselves without the intent to die. As kids get older, the number rises: 23% of teenagers and 38% of college students and young adults report self-injury. Rates of NSSI among adolescents who require hospitalization are even higher, with up to 40% of inpatients having NSSI. The behavior appears to decline after age 24, and yet self-injury occurs in about 4% of adults in the United States.

> ## MOST COMMON TYPES OF SELF-INJURY
>
> Research by Janice Whitlock (2010) and many others shows that skin cutting is the most common (70–90%) form of self-injury, followed by head banging or hitting (21%–44%), and then burning (15%–35%). The reason that these numbers add up to more than 100% is that some people engage in more than one form of NSSI. NSSI by way of cutting the skin most often occurs on the wrists and arms, stomach, ankles, thighs, and in women, the breasts.

Could your child be engaging in nonsuicidal self-injury? Here are some signs to look for:

- Scars that indicate healed cuts or burns.
- Wearing long sleeves and long pants where the child often wore short sleeves or shorts, to hide scars.
- Finding razors or other cutting implements in their clothes or room.
- Observing an uptick in bruises or other "injuries" that cannot be explained.

Why would anyone who has been repeatedly sexually abused start harming herself? Adolescents tell us that the most common reasons they self-injure are:

1. To reduce intense negative emotions, such as anger, guilt, shame, the fear of being abandoned, and unbearable depression.
2. Because the experience of self-loathing is paired with thoughts, such as that they are terrible people, toxic to others, or deserve to be punished.
3. When they experience dissociation or numbing, as a way of feeling something rather than the emptiness that comes from feeling nothing.

These types of distress are common in affected youth. Although we don't fully understand how it works, research shows that NSSI is a highly effective way to regulate or control intense emotions and unwanted thoughts. If you discover that your child has been self-injuring, it's important to know that she's doing it to ease the types of internal distress that result from the abuse. It's just as critical, however, for you and your child to understand that *NSSI may work in the short run but is an ineffective emotion-regulation strategy in the long run,* as Kayla discovered. And even if it provides temporary relief, self-injury does prevent children and teens from learning longer-term and healthier coping mechanisms.

> Self-injury can temporarily ease emotional pain, but resorting to it prevents sexual abuse victims from learning healthy ways to cope and heal.

Suicidality

Even though youth who self-injure aren't trying to kill themselves, and in most cases the cutting or other injury isn't seriously harmful, research shows that people who self-injure are at high risk for suicide. Specifically NSSI is associated with a fivefold increase in the likelihood of a suicide attempt within the next 6 months after self-injury in adolescents receiving outpatient psychiatric treatment. In teenagers not receiving psychiatric treatment, NSSI is associated with a sevenfold increase in risk for future suicide attempts. Thus the frequency of self-injury matters. In one study by Daniel Zahl and Keith Hawton in 2004, 4.7% of people who repeatedly self-injured died by suicide, compared with 1.9% of those who had only one episode of NSSI over the 15 years of the study. These findings don't mean that if your child is cutting she is probably also thinking about suicide, but it's important to consider the possibility, and any signs of NSSI are strong signals to seek professional help.

> Take any discovery of self-harm or reckless behavior seriously from the start—self-destructive behavior tends to escalate and therefore demands immediate professional intervention.

As Kayla's writings from the month before she entered McLean reveal, she felt besieged by PTSD symptoms, including nightmares, periods of dissociation, anger and irritability, pervasive feelings of worthlessness, and a great deal of ruminative thinking and guilt related to Daniel:

May 27, 2007 (age 16)

Dear God,

    Well, another week has come and passed. You'd think that in light of all that has happened my mother and I would be united, but somehow we manage to be pushed even further away from each other. She wants me to take care of myself—I'm supposed to find my own counselor—but if she feels the slightest bit out-of-control she says that I'm under the age of 18 and she's the boss. It's funny how the cards seem to go both ways for her.

    I miss him. I tell myself not to, and I tell myself that I hate him, but deep down I know he's right and I'm wrong. Maybe in the beginning I was not a whore, but I am now. No one knows the real me. No one knows how I feel or think, only you. But he knew me the best. He still does. He knows that one day this is all gonna catch up to me.

    My thoughts are twisted. One minute I love him and the next I hate him. I know now that he never loved me, but all I can see is his face. I try so hard to block it out it makes me start hurting.

    He's in my dreams telling me to call him—he misses me; he wants to talk to me. In my head at practice telling me what to do. Telling me what to wear again. He is there in my mind always like a ghost. God, sometimes I'm glad he's still telling me what to do; other times I want to scream.

    I get so angry lately. Even at Brian. I know it's because of him. He wants me to hate Brian, but I love him. I know I do. The way I feel with him—safe. He feels sorry for me, and I don't want that. Even though Daniel's not here he still finds a way to torture me.

    Love Always,
    Kayla

Is your child experiencing suicidal thoughts? See the warning signs in the box on page 157.

> Because of our inability to predict which threats will lead to a suicide attempt and which won't, any statement that a child or teen is thinking about suicide *must* be taken seriously.

During the period before Kayla was finally persuaded by those around her to accept expert help, she continued to battle on her own with serious symptoms that included almost daily preoccupations with suicide. In the weeks leading up to her McLean admission and despite the concerns and overtures

SIGNS THAT A CHILD
MAY BE HAVING THOUGHTS OF SUICIDE

There's no foolproof test that can predict suicide, but there are some warning signs that should alert a parent to be concerned and to contact a mental health provider.

- *Excessive sadness or mood swings:* Mood swings that appear to come from nowhere and episodes of unexpected rage.
- *Hopelessness:* Expressions of feelings that things in the person's life are never going to get better.
- *Withdrawal and isolation:* Insistence on being alone or avoidance of friends, particularly if this is new behavior.
- *Dangerous or self-injurious behavior:* Sudden reckless driving, increased use of drugs or alcohol, and particularly self-injury through cutting, punching, or burning.
- *Researching methods:* Spending time researching how to commit suicide, typically online.
- *Threatening suicide:* Up to 75% of people considering suicide give someone who is relationally close some warning sign. This is not a reliable indicator, however, as in most cases the threat of suicide does not mean that the person will follow through.

from teammates and coaches, Kayla still used her journal as the only place where she fully divulged her ongoing desperation:

June 11, 2007 (age 16)

Dear God,

Well, I've been in Boston for a while now. I start my new job tomorrow. I wish I could write how I really feel right now, but to be honest I don't really know. Sometimes I hate it here. Sometimes I love it.

I don't think Jimmy likes me. I don't think anyone here likes me. I think about killing myself still. I think about just hanging myself from the ceiling fan in my room. Every time I look at it, that's what I think. And then he pops in my head and says don't do it. Be strong. Be a fighter. And I want to scream at him. Fuck you. You're not a fighter; you're a coward. That's why you're lying to everyone about us.

God, I want someone to hate so bad. Someone to blame. And then I realize there's no one to hate but myself. Nobody made me this way. This is just how I turned out. I'm a bitch. There is no reason I'm a slut. There is no reason I am the way I am. I am because I make myself. I make myself lie. I make myself hateful. It's my own doing. I don't deserve forgiveness. I don't deserve love. I don't deserve anyone or anything. I'm sorry God. I know I don't deserve your forgiveness but I ask it anyway. Please forgive me and help me, God.

Love always,
Kayla

Other Dangerous Behavior

Although self-injury and suicidality are not included as criteria for a diagnosis of PTSD, research efforts led by our colleagues Randy Auerbach and Matt Nock in 2014 at Harvard Medical School have found a strong and consistent relationship between childhood abuse and later serious NSSI and suicidal behavior. These behaviors are considered to be part of a group of emotion regulation difficulties characteristic of complex PTSD. Other researchers have found that, beyond the disorders of PTSD and complex PTSD, these victims are vulnerable to developing severe anxiety, phobias, and perhaps most critical in terms of the victim's ultimate survival, problems with depression and severe substance use over time.

Obviously substance use is a risky behavior, and victims of prolonged sexual abuse may also behave impulsively in a variety of other ways, taking risks they would not have taken before and seeking out interactions with people or social settings that could endanger them. This behavior often takes the form of promiscuous sexual involvements, aggressive encounters, ignoring personal safety issues, such as driving too fast or without a seatbelt, and involvement in impulsive drug use in social settings.

Let's leave no room for doubt here: *The risks to a child's ongoing safety when the child has undergone long-term victimization by a sexual abuser who was in a position of trust and power relative to the child are very high. Even if you don't know the extent of your child's internal distress, any dangerously erratic behavior calls for finding a professional with expertise whom your child can talk to.*

We know that a child who displays the kinds of behavior or mood swings after revealing abuse that Kayla describes so vividly is not likely to get better without professional help that targets the symptoms of PTSD and more. We also know that several forms of CBT can be used effectively with children, adolescents, and adults to help them learn effective strategies for managing the reminders of their past traumatic experiences so they can avoid resorting to dangerous behaviors. The same treatments can target the emotional distress of shame and guilt; the low self-esteem and the distorted perceptions of themselves, the perpetrator, and the world that victims experience; and the problems with relationships and daily functioning. We discuss these treatments later in the chapter, but the first step toward receiving them is to get an expert assessment.

GETTING A THOROUGH ASSESSMENT OF THE CHILD'S PROBLEMS

As we said in Chapter 4, when you first learn that your child has been abused, you may decide to consult your pediatrician, family health care practitioner, or internist. Although many children who have survived trauma find it difficult to have a physical exam, it is generally a good idea to have one because there are medical conditions such as diabetes or thyroid conditions that can complicate the treatment by causing symptoms like anxiety. Also if medications are going to be recommended as part of the treatment plan, they can affect heart rate, blood pressure, and liver tests.

Kayla's memories of having a physical exam and a gynecological exam underscore why preparing the child or teen for what will be involved in an evaluation and treatment is so critical:

Aside from the interviews and questioning from the police, one thing my mother felt was necessary right away was to have a physical exam by an OB/GYN. While I was not subjected to a rape kit or any kind of physical exam by the police, what I did undergo was my first appointment with a gynecologist in a very traumatic setting.

I was 16 and my mom took me for an emergency appointment. The doctor was a man, which made it feel even scarier. My mother explained the situation to him and asked that he test me for every-thing. I remember crying and trying not to let the tears slide down my face. I couldn't look the doctor in the eye. I still felt dirty and scared. My mom stayed in the room for the whole procedure. The doctor was very patient and explained everything to my mom. They would test for all STDs, and I remember him saying something about AIDS. My hymen was broken, but everything else seemed normal. They discussed birth control and if I should be on it. My mother felt it was a good idea. But I felt as if I wasn't even in the room. It was as if I wasn't there. The bedside manner was as if I was a child and I remember feeling like I was a lab rat in a test tube. Once the procedure was over he explained to my mom they would get the results in about a week and wrote a prescription for a birth control pill. Then he said that I was free to go. That day I went home and went to my room and stared at the ceiling for what must have been hours. I wondered when it was going to end. If it would ever end. If I would ever feel clean again.

Your pediatrician or other health care practitioner can also refer you to a mental health professional who can assess your child for trauma symptoms. Once it's clearer that your child needs treatment, the next step is finding an appropriate therapist. Here is a guide to finding such a therapist.

Finding a Therapist

A therapist is any independently licensed mental health provider, such as a psychologist, psychiatrist, social worker, or licensed mental health counselor.

Checklist for Identifying a Qualified Therapist

• *Not all therapists are experienced in treating people who have experienced a trauma.* Don't assume that being a psychologist means the practitioner is an expert in PTSD. Specifically ask if a particular therapist has experience in treating trauma.

• *Depending on where you live, the availability of a trauma expert may be limited.* Certainly in larger urban areas, and particularly those with teaching hospitals, there will be clinicians who not only are experienced in treating trauma but also use the latest evidence-based treatments for PTSD. Typically these treatments involve more than simply talking about the past and include a behavioral component or the learning of new skills. Evidence-based therapies include CBT, prolonged exposure therapy (PE), prolonged exposure therapy with DBT (DBT PE), cognitive processing therapy (CPT), and eye movement desensitization and reprocessing (EMDR) therapy. In response to the demand that all military veterans receive PTSD treatment, websites like *www.talkspace.com* are now available to ensure remote access to expert care for people who do not have specialists in their area.

- *Not all therapists accept all insurance plans.* You may want to call your insurance company to see if the therapist you've found is covered by your insurance plan. If not, you can ask for the names of providers who are covered. Or if the therapist is not covered by your plan, you can ask what your out-of-pocket cost will be. Alternatively sometimes insurance companies will cover an out-of-network provider if they don't have a specialist in their network.

- *If you are in the fortunate position to have more than one choice of therapist, you might want to interview the various therapists to see who would be a better fit* with regard to communication style, schedule, office location, and other factors.

- *Most professions have a licensing board that keeps records of a therapist's professional conduct and legal history,* and in many states these records are available online. Legal judgments against a therapist don't necessarily indicate that the therapist is incompetent, unethical, or unprofessional, but you may want to clarify the nature of the circumstances, particularly if there have been concerns about boundary violations.

Questions to Ask the Therapist

Once you've identified a therapist and established logistics like billing, the answers to certain questions will be helpful in making your final decision:

- How do you protect confidentiality?
- How long is each session?
- If my child is in a crisis, would I be able to reach you?
- What is your vacation coverage?
- How will we monitor progress?
- How will you interface with my child's pediatrician/school/prescriber to coordinate treatment?

BEFORE STARTING IN THERAPY

If the child is at school, you may wish to consider including the school counselors among those who are notified about the abuse so that the school is aware. While school accommodations can help some victims establish a sense of safety, for others notifying school personnel will feel like a further violation of the victim's privacy and thus increase her distress and feelings of vulnerability. As with all postdisclosure matters, the critical guideline here is to talk with your child and make sure that she both understands and has a chance to weigh the pros and cons of all interventions being considered on her behalf.

Finally, it's important to prepare the child for treatment.

- Reassure the child that she will retain control over her own fate, but ask her for a commitment to try it.
- Explain that she may continue to shift between feeling better and feeling worse for a time on the road to recovery.
- Underscore the idea that her safety—from the perpetrator as well as from self-destructive impulses she may have been having—will always be the first priority of her treatment (and for you, her parent).
- Tell her that an ongoing goal of treatment will be to teach her skills that will help her deal with the disturbing thoughts and feelings that she has been dealing with for so long and that may be even worse now that her ordeal has been revealed (the subject of Chapter 7).
- Assure her that the goal of recovery is not just treating the symptoms of trauma but helping her return to the life she had and deserves, with all of its hopes and dreams.

What to Expect from an Assessment

If you are having your child evaluated by a psychologist or other mental health professional after a sexual abuse disclosure, you should expect to receive the following information when the assessment is completed:

- A detailed review of what type of abuse the child experienced, including the length and severity and the relationship to the perpetrator.
- A review of the disclosure process, including the status of any

mandated reports to child protection and any pending court or criminal complaints.

- A review of current safety at home and elsewhere to assess ongoing risks of maltreatment/abuse.

- Risk assessment, including any self-destructive or suicidal behaviors that the child is currently having or has engaged in.

- A review of other symptoms, including of the child's mood, eating, substance use, and involvement in any high-risk behaviors (including sexual behaviors).

- A review of the child's mental status, including any problems with dissociation, and an overall assessment of the child's thoughts and beliefs about the abuse.

- A review of whether the child meets the full criteria for PTSD, as well as any other psychiatric disorders.

- A review of the child's functioning in school and elsewhere (sports, social situations, etc.).

- A review of treatment recommendations, including a proposed treatment plan for addressing any self-harming or suicidal behaviors.

- Recommendations for when and how to treat diagnosed PTSD, including medication options and therapy.

After being referred to McLean, Kayla came into the hospital voluntarily with the understanding that she would be able to do her judo training in the evenings.

She did not want medications to address her possible depression and PTSD symptoms, instead wanting to use the behavioral treatment skills we teach in order to try to learn how to deal with her existing self-destructive thoughts and feelings. Because of the fact that I (Dr. Aguirre) worked out with Kayla at judo, I did not participate directly in her case. Instead, I asked two trusted colleagues, a social worker and a psychiatrist who understood PTSD, to do a more thorough clinical interview and workup. In her initial psychiatric admission note of 6/25/07 my colleague wrote:

History and presenting problem:

Kayla is a 16-year-old female with a 4-year history of being sexually abused by her coach since age 12. She complains of depressed mood, reduced appetite, reduced concentration, hopelessness, suicidal ideation, insomnia, nightmares, flashbacks, and dissociative symptoms. She denies psychotic or anxiety symptoms.

Social:

Kayla grew up in Dayton, Ohio, with her mother and stepfather. She has an 8-year-old brother and a 12-year-old sister. Aiming for Olympics in 2008. Schooling—straight A's.

Past psychiatric history:

Recent contact with Boston Rape Crisis Center. Reports cutting 1 year ago. Reports history of anorexia and bulimia at age 12–13. Denies current eating-disordered symptoms. Tried Prozac in the past, but no longer taking it as did not feel it was effective.

Drug abuse: Denies

Mental Status Exam:

Kayla is a cooperative well-groomed female, with normal speech and avoidant eye contact. Her stated mood is "depressed" and her affect is depressed. She admits to passive thoughts of suicide, however has no plan or intent at this time. She denies homicidal ideation, auditory or visual hallucinations.

Diagnosis:

PTSD

Major depression

Plan:

Admit to the residential unit.

Review medications.

Start skills training in the DBT classroom to stabilize unsafe behaviors.

Identify skilled after-care provider.

These condensed notes give an idea of the scope of information that will be collected when a mental health professional first sees a patient. The goal is to render a diagnosis and prepare an initial treatment plan. In Kayla's case the practitioner at McLean determined that Kayla was suffering from PTSD plus depression, along with ongoing problems with managing distress via high-risk/high-stakes behaviors. This is why DBT skills training was at the center of her initial treatment plan. As described in more detail later, DBT is an adaptation of CBT that has strong research evidence for reducing symptoms of NSSI and suicidal thinking. DBT in adolescents is effective in reducing hospitalizations, suicidal ideation, NSSI, and treatment dropout and is the approach that we use in our residential treatment programs for initial stabilization.

The Symptom History

In Kayla's initial evaluation we also discovered that she was preoccupied with ruminative thoughts about her relationship with Daniel. Those thoughts in turn triggered the impulse to run away from everything, including life itself. Like many victims of similar abuse, Kayla felt guilty about prosecuting her abuser and also shamed by the realization that she didn't share in the rage and desire for revenge that was apparently uppermost in her mother's mind. This is why it's so critical to recognize that many aspects of a victim's story and thinking may still be largely undiscovered after disclosure, and that she may need specialized treatment to help her fully reveal, understand, and process all that she's been through.

Toward that end we typically ask clients who enter our programs and practices to talk with us or write what we refer to as a "symptom history," which amounts to a brief chronicle of problems that the adolescent can identify that brought her in for treatment. In her symptom history Kayla writes about her sexual abuse, her disclosure, and the turmoil of her everyday existence immediately before admission.

Produced almost immediately *after* her admission to McLean, Kayla's written account of her symptom history has been kept for over 10 years now because it reminds her of when she first was able to share her story—*all of her story*. Not the version that the police and her mother wanted to hear and not the version that people in her town, who knew of Daniel's arrest, speculated about. This was for Kayla the first chance to talk about her abuse, along with all the confusion, shame, longing, and despair that she had experienced. And it was an opportunity as well to take the risk to trust again and to let others, fellow residents and staff alike, bear witness to all that she had been through:

Symptom history For McLean Hospital upon Admission: 6/28/2007

At the age of 12 my mother and family physician decided I needed counseling. I was lashing out at my family. I didn't want to get out of bed and I was just generally depressed.

First of all let me just say that I just finished reading Tanya and Andi's symptom histories and let me just say I feel in no way shape or form do I deserve to be here. Here are two girls whose whole lives have been train wrecks and here I sit pitying myself. It just makes me realize how unjust the world is. And I don't even know these girls but I wish I could take away their pain. I wish that their lives had been different and that we had met in art class instead of the hospital. But since I'm here and they were strong enough to tell their stories I will do my best to tell mine.

I started judo at the age of 6. I wasn't very good but within a year I switched clubs and Daniel began coaching me. God he used to scare the shit out of me. He was always screaming at someone. Well after a while he became my world—or judo did. It's hard to separate the two. Nevertheless I ate breathed and lived for judo, for him. I remember wrestling with him at the hotels after tournament or clinging to him in the pool at the deep end. I was always a touchy-feely child. Things went on in that manner until I was 12 when he digitally penetrated me for the first time. I wasn't scared just confused and from there we went to sex which turned into him spending countless nights over at my house. I already loved him but every day it grew and grew until we were together—a couple.

I thought our relationship was normal back then—as normal as a secret can be. When we were alone things were good. Around other people he was different though. I was never good enough for him. So I trained harder. I quit school and started online school so I could train. I fought with everyone all the time and I couldn't stop. Before that my freshman year I lived with my grandparents for a little while because things at home got so bad.

Of course Daniel was there for me he always was and I was there for him. We were each other's support system. But after a while it became unhealthy. He was obsessive. If I even looked at a guy the wrong way he was down the back of my throat calling me a whore. That's just how he was though. I've always been heavy and he didn't let me forget it.

In April my world as I knew it came crashing down. I found out that Daniel had gone on a cruise with Mary, an old friend who he swore up and down was just his friend. So I ended it, or tried to.

When he cried I snapped. The next week we went down to Puerto Rico for a tournament. At this point we were not together. When we got down there he had a mental breakdown. He got drunk off his ass and I ended up taking care of him. I sent him home on an earlier flight, and tried to keep the team from falling apart.

A week later I competed at the US senior nationals. I had moved down a weight class so I had mostly just been focusing on making weight. I had been favored to win but that day ended up being the absolute worst day physically and emotionally of my life. I lost. Second place. My world was smashed into tiny pieces. All these months of hard work down the drain. No Pan Ams. No worlds. And it was all my fault. No one to blame but me. I couldn't blame Daniel. He wasn't out there losing the match for me.

On the ride home I was devastated. I was still in shock. Brian, my training partner just kept pushing and pushing me about what was wrong with me and Daniel and finally I cracked. I told him everything. And he had me call my mom who immediately meted out revenge. I told the police what they wanted to know. I came here even though I feel this is terrible timing to be away from judo.

The day of the restraining order hearing my mom packed me up and moved me to Boston. Since then I've been living on my own in every sense of the word. I do my own laundry, I work, I pay bills and rent. I cook my own food. I am a functioning adult, so to speak. I do get depressed and overwhelmed but I thought I could handle it in my own personal way and I clearly can't. So now I'm here and I'm going to make the best of it. And hopefully I come out of here having learned something.

And, as the rest of this book will show, she did.

PSYCHOTHERAPY FOR PTSD: WHAT ARE THE BEST CHOICES?

The goal of Kayla's treatment was for her to learn and then use DBT skills and principles to understand how running away and contemplating suicide were her solutions for momentarily escaping from the trauma-related thoughts, feelings, and beliefs instilled by her relationship with Daniel that remained too emotionally upsetting for her to manage. Gradually she came to appreciate that, despite the temporary emotional relief they provided, these were the very behaviors she would need to target for change to become stable enough to pursue her life goal of being an Olympic champion.

Skills-Focused and Exposure-Focused Phases of Treatment

Many different treatments are available to survivors of trauma, but most are based on the fundamental idea that safety—protection from NSSIs, suicidality, and risky behaviors—has to be established first. Trauma treatment involves teaching the child or teen skills for managing disturbing emotions and memories and avoiding the urges to harm herself or act in dangerously impulsive ways. This is generally thought of as *present-focused therapy* because it concentrates on helping the child or teen to learn and practice skills to help them become and remain stable right now. Only after this stability is achieved, and she has acquired the skills necessary to manage severe distress, will specific PTSD treatments that help in processing the past traumas be offered. These *past-focused treatments,* involving *exposure* to recollections of the trauma, help survivors to ultimately examine and challenge the specific trauma-related alterations in mood, beliefs, and behaviors that continue to cause them suffering.

In Kayla's case her safety remained precarious for some time after discharge and, given her rigorous training and travel schedule, she continued skills-focused DBT treatment on a weekly basis for quite some time, only gradually integrating a stronger focus on reconstructing and processing her past abuse.

Establishing Safety: DBT as a First-Phase Treatment

DBT, developed in 1993 by Dr. Marsha Linehan, combines skills training, emotional exposure, and cognitive modification strategies with mindfulness, validation, and acceptance practices. DBT was originally developed as a treatment for adults with dangerous levels of NSSI and suicidal behaviors and more recently has been adapted to help adolescents with multiple problem behaviors characterized by severe emotional dysregulation, NSSI, and suicidal behaviors.

People undergoing DBT skills training learn how to be mindfully aware of their emotions and let them pass as emotions do naturally, to use various methods to tolerate distress that are not self-destructive, to change their emotional response in taxing situations, and more. They learn to challenge negative automatic thoughts and distorted beliefs that whatever situation they are in is hopeless and simply has to be escaped.

In DBT skills training Kayla began to realize that when the judo mat at practice brought back images of Daniel she would immediately become flooded with feelings of sadness, guilt, and shame and, when these feelings became intolerable, would resort to running away, fighting, or thinking about dying—anything really to shift the focus away from her unbearable, trauma-related distress. She then learned DBT skills for how to tolerate this distress without obeying these urges, for how to manage crises, and for how to accept her emotions. As was true for Kayla, it takes time to learn these skills, and DBT can often feel like a one-step-forward, two-steps-back process. Recovery is rarely linear, but parents and other supportive adults and peers can help the victim stick with it, as those in Kayla's network did. Some of the commitment strategies we use include:

- Comparing the pros and cons of quitting therapy versus the pros and cons of continuing therapy.
- Using the devil's advocate technique, whereby the person is asked "Why not quit?" to strengthen the person's commitment and increase her sense of control and autonomy.
- Asking the person if she has ever made a commitment that she stuck to and how this present commitment matches up to previous ones.

During her first days at McLean, Kayla continued to make considerable progress on expanding her symptom history, learning to apply DBT skills, and gaining a better understanding of the functions that her self-destructive thoughts and behaviors served. Realizing that without professional help her self-destructive behaviors would likely continue to recur and threaten her Olympic dreams, Kayla made the commitment to continue working with a therapist on an outpatient basis, where the focus was on stopping the cycle of emotional distress, escape, and avoidance that had brought her into the hospital.

However, this increased awareness and improved control was coupled with the quandary faced almost universally by child sexual abuse survivors: "How, if I give up running away from the recollections and reminders of what happened to me, will I ever be able to make sense of, live with, and accept the awful reality of my abuse?"

The short answer we give to this common question is that it's possible not only to establish personal safety but also to take a look back at the abuse to understand, rather than try to outrun, the impact of these traumatic childhood experiences. In the context of a safe, therapeutic relationship, victims of childhood sexual abuse can deconstruct and reprocess their core trauma-related beliefs and emotions, recognizing that it's the unhelpful beliefs and unjustified emotions related to their abuse that continue to drive the cycle of unbearable distress, flight, and evasion. This reexposure to childhood abuse experiences in therapy may in fact be essential for many victims to make a full recovery, so it's critical to understand what the existing options are for targeted PTSD treatment and when it's appropriate to seek this type of help.

Guidelines issued by a variety of professional and governmental organizations that issue recommendations for PTSD treatment based on up-to-date scientific appraisals, as reported in 2013 by Stephanie Schneider and colleagues at the Center for Pediatric Traumatic Stress at Children's Hospital of Philadelphia, unanimously support CBT as the most effective treatment for PTSD. A majority also recommend EMDR (see page 174).

> Research has shown that CBT is the most effective treatment for PTSD.

CBT treatments for PTSD typically include a number of standard components, consisting of:

- Psychoeducation, which teaches both an individual and the family about PTSD.
- Skills training for effective mood regulation.
- Exposure to elements of the trauma.
- Cognitive restructuring of emotions and beliefs related to the trauma.

Of these components, *exposure* and *cognitive restructuring* are thought to be the most essential elements involved in change and are typically included as central aspects in most, if not all, CBT-based treatments for PTSD.

Exposure is a technique in behavior therapy that involves the planned introduction of the patient to a feared situation, in the absence of any real danger, so the person can overcome the emotional distress triggered by that situation. For sexual abuse survivors, exposures are typically aimed at both memories of the abuse and present-day situations that are avoided because of their association with the past trauma; an example of this is Kayla becoming triggered emotionally at the sight of a judo mat reminiscent of her time with Daniel.

Cognitive restructuring helps patients learn to identify and challenge irrational or unhelpful thoughts so that they can eliminate them.

The following are currently accepted evidence-based therapies that use each of these approaches.

Exposure-Based Treatments for PTSD

A large number of studies have been conducted on a form of CBT that is primarily exposure based. In this type of therapy survivors receive the support they need to reexperience a traumatic event by recalling, rewriting, and/or retelling in detail what happened to them during the initial traumatic experience. This allows them to process problematic emotions like guilt, shame, and fear and beliefs such as "This happened to me because I deserved it" that are connected to the original traumatic experience. There is strong evidence that exposure of this kind can help to decrease PTSD symptoms.

Prolonged exposure (PE), developed by Edna Foa at the University of Pennsylvania and her colleagues, has received the most empirical support among exposure-based treatments. In PE, the patient undergoes exposure to memories of trauma along with exposure to current situations that trigger symptoms because they're associated with the original trauma. PE usually takes 8 to 15 weekly sessions, so treatment lasts about 3 months, and it includes daily homework between sessions that involves both listening to tapes of sessions and practicing exposure tasks. Sessions are typically 1.5 hours each and delivered in an individual therapy format. Licensed mental health professionals can obtain PE training by attending online or in-person workshops and can also obtain advanced PE certification. The Association for Behavioral and Cognitive Therapies (ABCT) is a good resource for finding a trained PE provider (*www.findcbt.org/xFAT*).

Is prolonged exposure a good option for your child or teen? In child, teen, and adult survivors of sexual abuse, rape, and combat, PE produced a significantly greater reduction in PTSD symptoms than present-centered, skills-based therapies or non-evidence-based treatments alone. Notably, there is also an adolescent version, PE-A, which includes all identified practice elements considered essential for the treatment of youth with PTSD, including contact and involvement with nonoffending caregivers.

However, you may encounter clinicians who are hesitant to prescribe PTSD therapies, particularly exposure, before being assured that the survivor has achieved a specific, enduring level of stability. This caution is understandable, but it can also delay treatment unduly, without a plan for actively providing skills training to victims of abuse so they could in fact become stable enough for treatment. Fortunately, research is being conducted to make exposure and other targeted trauma/PTSD treatments available much sooner, in a safe manner, so that victims get the help they need as soon as possible. Also, a 2011 review article on treatments for complex PTSD, by Marylene Cloitre and colleagues, published in the *Journal of Traumatic Stress,* indicated that 84% of 50 expert clinicians endorsed a phase-based or sequenced approach as a first-line treatment for this.

Recently, we've seen that individuals with severe forms of PTSD and life-threatening behaviors can tackle the exposure to past abuse recollections more immediately than first thought. Dr. Melanie Harned from the University of Washington has pioneered an outpatient treatment based on combining DBT and PE in sequence (mentioned earlier), and this approach has been shown to significantly reduce PTSD symptoms in women with co-occurring PTSD and borderline personality disorder (BPD) and histories of serious NSSI and suicidal behaviors. Currently, this treatment requires clients to have 8 weeks without NSSI or suicidal behaviors and to meet a number of other tests of their capacity before beginning the exposure-based work.

Dr. Bohus and his colleagues, working in an intensive residential setting in Germany, have also demonstrated that, following an initial period of skills acquisition and practice in learning to manage dissociative urges, exposure work can be started safely within 4 weeks of admission and with the treatment milieu acting to reinforce skill use and promote analysis of

> Promising new treatments allow victims a faster route to recovery by starting exposure very soon after teaching them skills for maintaining safety and abstaining from self-destructive behavior.

occurrences of unsafe behaviors. To date this approach (DBT-PTSD) has been used successfully with both female teenagers (ages 15+) and adult women with BPD and trauma histories, and it's worth considering in the future as a treatment option for even younger adolescents.

Cognitive Approaches

CBT approaches that prioritize *cognitive interventions* have also been found to be helpful in research reviewed by Anke Ehlers and colleagues at the University of Oxford. Among these approaches, two stand out.

Cognitive processing therapy (CPT), developed in the 1980s by Duke University professor Patricia Resick and her colleagues, is one of the most well-researched cognitive approaches for PTSD treatment in adult survivors and has been expanded more recently for use with adolescents as well as adults, although research support on the developmentally adapted CPT manual (D-CPT) is in its first stages of development. The primary focus of CPT is first identifying and then challenging and modifying unhelpful beliefs related to past trauma. Versions both with and without a written exposure component are available. CPT usually takes 12 weekly sessions, so treatment lasts about 3 months. Sessions are 60 to 90 minutes each, and homework is assigned to the client between sessions. CPT can be done individually, where you meet one-to-one with a provider, and can also be done in a group, with one or two providers and about 6 to 10 other people who also have PTSD. Providers can be found through the International Society for Traumatic Stress Studies website (*www.istss.org/find-a-clinician.aspx*).

Trauma-focused CBT (TF-CBT) may be more suitable for survivors of sexual abuse because rigorous testing over many years has shown that it can decrease PTSD, depressive symptoms, and trauma-related emotions and beliefs in both children and teens when compared to other non-CBT interventions. The TF-CBT model, developed by Judith Cohen and her colleagues, comprises nine key components now considered critical to the treatment, particularly of younger children who have experienced childhood abuse. The components are represented by the acronym PRACTICE:

- **P**sychoeducation
- **R**elaxation skills
- **A**ffective (emotion) modulation (regulation) skills

- Cognitive coping skills
- Trauma narrative and processing
- In vivo exposure (exposure to current triggering situations)
- Conjoint child–parent sessions
- Enhancing safety skill development

TF-CBT, typically delivered in 12–16 sessions, is appropriate for children and adolescents ages 3–18 years, and includes the direct involvement of the youth's parent or other caregiver in treatment. Mental health professionals can receive additional training in this approach (see *https://tfcbt.musc.edu*); when seeking treatment of this kind it is important to ask about the therapist's training and length of time practicing TF-CBT.

Eye Movement Desensitization and Reprocessing Therapy (EMDR)

Patients receiving EMDR are instructed to do imaginal exposure to a trauma while engaging in specific eye movements known as saccadic movements. A typical EMDR session lasts from 60 to 90 minutes, but the number of sessions deemed necessary depends on the type and severity of previous trauma and other factors. EMDR is thought to work by having the patient recall the distressing events while diverting attention from their emotional consequences, which makes it somewhat similar to PE. Although the American Psychiatric Association lists EMDR as an effective treatment for both acute and chronic PTSD, its mechanisms are not well understood, and there is less research to support this approach than other evidenced-based treatment. It also hasn't been studied extensively in children and teens, and there is a consensus that more research is needed to determine how effective EMDR is compared to other evidence-based treatments. In addition more research is needed to determine whether the benefits last. Information about finding practitioners can be found through the EMDR International Association (*www.emdria.org*).

Acceptance and Commitment Therapy (ACT) and the Neurosequential Model of Therapeutics (NMT)

A more recently developed type of behavioral therapy, ACT has shown some efficacy for patients with PTSD according to research by Susan

Orsillo and Sonja Batten. ACT focuses on reducing avoidance and preoccupations with unhelpful thinking and supports patients in participating in activities consistent with their personal values. Kayla, as an example, although not treated with ACT specifically, believes strongly that it was the return to her core value of hard work and her goal of being an Olympian that helped with her post-McLean recovery (discussed in greater detail in Chapter 7). And taking a more developmentally informed approach, Dr. Bruce Perry has developed a model (NMT) that, rather than focusing on the implementation of any one specific therapeutic approach over another, focuses on identifying the key systems and areas in a child's brain that have been impacted by adverse developmental experiences, and then using this individual information to select and sequence intervention strategies as well as enrichment and educational activities. To date, the results for the use of NMT across a number of clinical settings has been quite positive, and more investigations of treatment efficacy are currently under way.

Medication

There has been great interest over the years in exploring the role of medications in the treatment of PTSD. Currently it's unclear what types of medication are most helpful for individuals with this diagnosis, but CBT has consistently proven more effective than pharmacotherapy alone and should be considered as the first-line treatment for PTSD, either alone or in conjunction with appropriate medications.

THE ROAD TO RECOVERY

Once discharged and feeling safer, Kayla had to figure out how to prioritize ongoing treatment within a daily schedule of demanding athletic training. Survivors understandably want to resume important activities, as Kayla did, but it can be a challenge to treat residual trauma symptoms outside of an intensive treatment program. The risk of returning to unsafe behaviors while still learning to manage emotional distress is high. Even when an individual no longer meets the full criteria for PTSD, trauma reminders and cues can trigger increased distress at unexpected times, and that distress, in turn, can lead to a relapse of life-threatening symptoms. Your child might struggle with persistent sadness, a sense of being different from others, preoccupations with the fate of her perpetrator, difficulty trusting people in her life, and difficulties with making and keeping both friendships and romantic relationships. Therefore besides present-focused treatments aimed at establishing safety, like DBT, and specific PTSD treatments to allow for the processing of the past trauma, your child may need help reconnecting with others and then reestablishing a sense of mastery and empowerment in everyday life. Judy Herman, in her seminal book *Trauma and Recovery* (1992), talks about how, within the therapeutic relationship, survivors of abuse can once again establish the safety that allows for "remembrance and mourning" and promotes the necessary reconnection with everyday life. Reestablishing trust, meaningful relationships, and achievable goals is thus an ongoing challenge for sexual abuse victims and can take considerable time and effort on the part of your child, your family, and those in the child's support network.

What does this entail for you as a parent and for your child? It entails helping a child who is no longer in therapy and has a therapist for support to figure out how to once again make friendships and confide in others when for so long she often has lived an isolative, secretive existence. This requires testing who can be trusted and facing fears about what others may know about her abuse and whether they will understand. Sometimes it involves reaching out to organizations dedicated to helping other victims. Kayla describes how her mother steered her to the Boston Area Rape Crisis Center:

I did visit them [BARCC] when I first arrived in Boston. My mother sought them out to try and find a therapist and possibly some kind of support network for me outside of judo. This was probably right before I was hospitalized at McLean. I only went once, but years later I returned and was honored as one of their champions of change after sharing my story.

There are many routes to survival and recovery, as Kayla describes in the next two chapters. In Chapter 7 she discusses how CSA victims frequently develop a generalized sense of inadequacy and helplessness and need to once again establish personal goals and find ways to master them effectively.

For Kayla, maintaining a commitment to therapy so that she could move on with her life, without compromising her athletic goals or her emotional stability, meant agreeing to outpatient DBT treatment at McLean. Therapy was reinforced within the respectful and encouraging relationships she had formed with the Pedros, her teammates, and concerned family members, all of whom continued to stick close and cheer Kayla on:

My grandparents remained the biggest role models in my life. Both my Mimi and Poppy (Mom's parents) and my Mamaw and Papaw (Dad's parents) were my rocks. I grew up 5 minutes away from both of them, and from the time I can remember I always loved spending time with them. With my parents suffering in the aftermath of the abuse and sometimes unable to hide their anger or talk to me with a clear mind, my grandparents remained strong pillars that were a constant in my life I knew I could trust. They were supportive, understanding, and nonjudgmental and always made me feel loved. I cannot remember a time where I have ever been upset with them and vice versa. They have always been the people I wanted to make most proud, and that feeling of wanting to make them proud has led me down a good path.

In Kayla's estimation, it was these ongoing real-life supports that were critical, along with the professional help and treatment she received, in paving the way for her eventual recovery and success:

So many people ask me all the time how I made it through. How I got to be where I am today. What makes me special? How did I survive? And every time the answer is the same. Every time I tell them: It wasn't me. It was the people around me.

When I moved to Boston, I was a mess. I was an emotional car wreck. Rock bottom is putting it lightly. But Jimmy and Big Jim changed all that. They didn't allow me to stay in rock bottom. And neither did my teammates.

They picked me up when I was down. They held my hand on the bad days. They gave me tough love. They refused to let me quit on myself, on my life. They were my rocks and my saviors. Most importantly, they believed in me when nobody else did.

So that's it. That's the secret. If you're ever in trouble, find yourself a Pedro and hold on tight to them.

It isn't always easy to cheer on an abuse survivor, who has to constantly struggle to overcome the aftermath of trauma, as Kayla attests:

The Pedros were, like, "No, fuck you, you're getting out of bed, you're going to lifting. No, you're gonna go back to school. No, you're going to go to therapy . . ." It was tough love from the Pedros, but it was also survival. It was, like, well, I have to work or I'm not gonna be able to pay my rent, and then I'm going to get kicked out.

And it wasn't just survival—it was the daily structure, which provides a distraction from emotional triggers and disturbing memories that helped Kayla move forward, toward the Olympics and recovery:

I hate the term "power through," but I was waking up every morning for training, and then I was going to school, and then I was going to judo after school, and I was working. Structure was huge for me. If I didn't have that and I had just been allowed to wallow in my own self-loathing it's hard to say where I would have wound up. But it wouldn't have been in a good place. And certainly it wouldn't have been on top of the podium.

With time Kayla began to use her outpatient DBT treatment as a springboard for gradual, planned exposures to her past trauma in the form of thinking, writing, and talking about how her abuse started, progressed, and eventually ended in disclosure. And as part of this exposure work, Kayla took the important step of daring to look back at her journal entries from the more recent past—entries that became the vehicle for the emotional processing work she had to undertake with her therapist, work that was no doubt necessary for her full recovery.

Through a reexamination of her journal writings and a reconstruction of past trauma, Kayla realized that she had unwittingly created a chronicle of her grooming and molestation at Daniel's hands, and that this narrative could possibly form the basis of a cautionary tale that might help others avoid, or at least shorten, the suffering of child sexual abuse. This realization further fueled Kayla's determination that she would one day feel strong enough to share her story with the world—a determination that intensified as Kayla returned to the gym and her long-held dream of becoming the first American to win an Olympic gold medal in judo. In Kayla's own words:

It was such a hard thing to trust again, to love again after sexual abuse. It's not something you can ever do alone.

I still saw a therapist every week. If it weren't for therapy, if it wasn't for the people that I surrounded myself with, I never would have learned to love again, I never would have learned to trust again, I never would have opened up.

If you're a survivor, it's something that it takes a long time to bring back out. And it starts with sharing your story.

And at McLean and in DBT they talk about your "mastery" ... judo was my mastery. It was my one place I could still be a kid and where I could achieve something through hard work and determination. It was a part of my life that I did not want to be ruined for me because of what had happened, and as I fought back on the mat I gradually regained my self-confidence and fought back against my past as well ... judo restored my belief in myself ... it made me feel good about myself again.

Kayla realized that many personal challenges lay ahead, emotional as well as athletic, challenges that she would have to face on her road to recovery. She was right that her suffering at this point was far from over and it would, in fact, take almost another year before she was able to stop self-injuring and was no longer plagued by frequent thoughts of suicide. Ongoing treatment, support from others close to her, structure in her daily life, and the setting and mastery of personal goals ultimately made up the formula for her recovery and eventual success—a formula that Kayla hopes will help others who have been hurt in childhood.

7

From Victim to Survivor

We cautioned at the beginning of Chapter 5 that those who care for children who have been victims of sexual abuse should not expect their suffering to end when the abuse ends. We must add here that the repercussions of chronic sexual abuse also don't end when the child or teen is stable enough to tackle PTSD symptoms directly through treatments like those discussed in Chapter 6. In fact, the handprint of chronic abuse can last for months and even years after professional help is sought. Just ask the survivors. Virtually all of them will tell you that they needed to use every professional and nonprofessional support they could find to keep moving forward with their recovery. Kayla captures this reality in her own words:

> What can I say that hasn't already been said about how important it is to have a support system around you. Pillars of strength and confidence. The Pedros were that for me. Team FORCE was that for me. I can honestly say I wouldn't be who I am today if it weren't for them. They changed my life—they saved my life.
>
> It wasn't all at once. It wasn't boom—you move to Boston and you're all better. But it was in the little moments. The first time I laughed after disclosing was at Chili's after training where we all went for the bottomless queso. The first time I felt good about myself again was when Big Jim saw me throwing someone during sparring and just simply said, "good throw . . . good throw." The first time I talked to my teammates about my past they didn't really know what to say—but they didn't have to say anything; it was enough

for them to listen. The first time I went to a tournament how they all stuck by me—like a mini shield of protection with Jimmy and Big Jim right by my side. The first time I smiled at a boy and didn't feel dirty, then ran home to tell all my teammates about it. Waking up at 5:00 A.M. to go to strength and conditioning on a Saturday and feeling so accomplished once it was done. Working 50 hours a week at a hardware store owned by my teammate's family. Teaching judo classes after school to kids who thought I was something special.

Slowly, ever so slowly turning judo—the thing that had almost ruined my life—back into my passion. One practice at a time. One day at a time. One breath at a time.

Sitting at Big Jim's lake house talking about my life and my goals and my possibilities. The tough love I needed. The guiding hand. My best friend, my father figure, my hero.

Traveling all over the world with my best friends. Seeing the Eiffel Tower. Watching the sun rise in Abu Dhabi. Climbing Mount Fuji. Winning, losing, learning, and growing. All the while building up the confidence to one day be who I was meant to be. All because of the people who shared that journey with me.

The trips, the trials, the ups the downs. The highs the lows. Big wins on the mat, big losses off. The memories of it all. The people who were there. Their faces are burned into my memory. And I truly felt as if every single one of them were on that podium with me in London.

People always ask me which medal I like better—Rio or London. Which one means more to me? And I always laugh and say—that's like picking a favorite child, I can't. But what I really want to say is this. Neither. It's not the medals that mean anything. It's the moments that culminated into those days that I cherish more than anything in life.

Clearly, Kayla's healing had only just begun by the time she was discharged from McLean and entered outpatient psychiatric treatment in the summer of 2007. At that time less was known about the importance of introducing targeted PTSD treatment as early as possible in a victim's recovery and, given Kayla's recent self-injury and suicidal thinking, she was referred for standard DBT treatment after discharge, with the primary goal of helping her use her newly acquired DBT skills to remain emotionally regulated and avoid any relapse back into self-destructive behaviors. Initially this therapy was completely present focused, and Kayla's PTSD symptoms were monitored only with the goal of minimizing their interference in her daily life. It was considered "too soon" for Kayla to begin the process of more thoroughly reconstructing and emotionally processing her past abuse.

Naturally it makes sense to address the intrusive symptoms of PTSD. Nightmares, unwanted memories of the abuse, and flashbacks, for example, are disruptive and can make it tough for a child to reclaim the normal life she once had. Unfortunately, though, tackling the surface symptoms is rarely enough. Chronic sexual abuse like Kayla's causes many underlying and pervasive disruptions to well-being that negatively affect the survivor's sense of identity, trust, and self-confidence. This is clear from Kayla's writings within the month after her discharge when, although actively engaged in an outpatient treatment, Kayla remained preoccupied on a daily basis with her past:

August 3, 2007 (6 weeks after leaving McLean)

Dear God,

I still cry every day. although I'm getting better and better at giving everyone a false sense of my happiness. I make sure it's in the shower or when I'm all alone.

I'm feeling more guilty every day. I can't even remember everything anymore, and it scares me because there's no known record of all the good times we had. So what if they just slip away into my memory forever? How will I know why I'm the person I am 10 years from now? Will I remember everything that's happened to me? Will I remember him? Will I remember the good or the bad, the beginning or the end? The happy times or the scary times? Will I remember the trial? The tournaments? Will I even remember at all?

I miss my old life. Everything is different these days.

Love Always,
Kayla

PERSISTENTLY MONITORING AND SUPPORTING THE CHILD

It's clear from this journal entry that Kayla is continuing to try to hide her inner turmoil from those who care about her. More often than not, there remains a cloak of secrecy and shame that can mask ongoing difficulties, difficulties the survivor frequently feels she should have "gotten past" once in treatment. Unless they are acknowledged or otherwise revealed, it's hard to alleviate them.

So what does it take to keep victims like Kayla moving effectively toward recovery, to make the transition from victim to survivor? From our work with survivors like Kayla we know that ongoing monitoring and support by parents, caregivers, and peers who interact with the child or teen on a daily basis is key. But the truth is that a full recovery takes time, and to keep the process on track, caring others need to notice ongoing difficulties and respond to them effectively.

> Well into treatment victims of CSA may try to hide symptoms that need to be addressed because they think they should be "over them" by now.

This is no easy or simple task, no matter how vigilant parents and caregivers try to be. This is why in Chapter 6 we stressed the advisability of ensuring that those who have been abused receive professional help for as long as a qualified practitioner believes it is needed. As a parent you may be well aware that your child still has nightmares about her abuse a year or two after it has ended. You might observe moodiness and irritability. But it can be much more difficult to recognize that a lot of perplexing behaviors are an expression of the persistent internal distress of complex PTSD and to respond to them in a way that keeps the child or teen on the path toward recovery:

- *Pay attention to problems with regulating emotions.* The anger, guilt, shame, sadness, and even related suicidal thoughts that have erupted after the extended silence during your child's abuse can remain difficult for your child to understand and manage. Without jumping at the slightest perplexing behavior, don't ignore lasting changes in your child's mood, shifts in temperament, or changes in her way of expressing emotions that leave you feeling unsure of how to help. Ask her how she's feeling and try to ensure that any problems are discussed with her mental health professionals. DBT and other treatments for PTSD can teach your child specific skills for emotion regulation.

- *Gently help your child stay in touch with her surroundings in the present.* When your child seems out of touch or forgets an incident that was notable to her in the past, resist responding with disbelief and insisting that of course your child must remember the same incident that everyone else in the family recalls. Refrain from confronting the child about what may appear to be excessive daydreaming from your perspective. Instead, gently help your child reconnect with the conversation as best she can by being both supportive and patient.

• *Validate the feelings of shame, guilt, and anger that may color your child's self-image.* Hearing child victims express feelings of being damaged or worthless can be very distressing to the parents who love them, but it's impossible to simply dissuade a child from feelings and beliefs that have developed as part of a childhood sexual trauma. All you can do is offer patience and understanding, validating that you understand that your child may feel different about himself from the way you see him while *not* validating this negative view of himself. Reinforce your belief that his view of himself will improve with time and often with treatment as well. Validating emotions is an important topic in DBT, and parents may benefit from learning more about this subject (see the Resources).

• *Resist the urge to correct your child's distorted perceptions of the perpetrator.* The complex web of feelings victims have toward the person who victimized them can last for a very long time and are often the most difficult aftermath of abuse for parents to deal with. Your feelings are likely more straightforward (except in some cases of incest, where the perpetrator is a trusted, loved member of the family). You're undoubtedly exceedingly angry and want the perpetrator to be punished to the fullest extent possible! While your feelings may be more straightforward toward the perpetrator, you may have complex and conflicting feelings about the abuse itself. For example, you too may feel shame and guilt along with your anger, badgering yourself about why you didn't know your child was being abused, how you could have entrusted the perpetrator with your child's safety, how you could have let your child down in this way. It's not easy to suppress these feelings when they are triggered by a child's sudden, surprising statement of concern or support—or even love—for the perpetrator, and parents may benefit from professional help for their own emotional struggles. The more you try to insert your own feelings and agenda into your child's recovery process, the less likely it will be that your child will be honest with you about her emotional turmoil and the more your child may work to hide positive or guilty feelings. Your child will need time and "permission" to mourn the loss of a relationship that may have been both hurtful *and* important to the child. The last thing you want to do is to make the child feel bad for having feelings that are at variance with yours. Respect the child's confusion and do not try to strong-arm the child in any way.

• *Help the child reestablish trusting relationships.* It's difficult to grasp how a developing young mind reconciles the trust he's been taught to have in adults who are caregivers or authorities with the physical and emotional brutality of sexual abuse. So it's no surprise that children and teens who have been betrayed in this way by a respected adult may take a long time to trust others to get close to them, to trust their own instincts about people, and to seek out companionship and intimacy with prudence instead of terror. While it is tempting to want to help your child make safe reconnections with the world, the best a parent can do is to give the child opportunities to engage with peers in a safe manner and to expect that this may take some time. Some tendency to isolate is to be expected, and as long as the child's need to be alone does not turn into any kind of extreme withdrawal (for example, refusing to go to school or go out at all), give your child time to gradually reconnect with others in a manner that he feels comfortable with and in control of. If, however, you observe your child engaging with people who are significantly older than she is or beginning to exhibit high-risk behaviors, such as socializing only with drugs or alcohol, it's time to set reasonable limits and seek additional professional help. Also beware of the possibility that a child who has suffered chronic abuse may be vulnerable to the advances of someone who appears to be a potential rescuer or protector. Professional treatment can help children develop healthy self-confidence and self-reliance, as well as confidence in their instincts, decision-making skills, and interpersonal skills that will help them form good relationships, gradually, as they mature.

• *Promote stability at home and get professional help with any changes in your child's core beliefs about herself and her world.* Core beliefs and values evolve throughout childhood and adolescence and form a foundation for a child's ability to find meaning in an often unpredictable world. A child's beliefs about the fairness of the world and the meaning of life and her values regarding how people should behave can become distorted by this devastating experience. When you see signs that your child's basic beliefs have been negatively affected by the abuse, she probably needs to talk through the dissonance between what she believed before the abuse and what may have become long-held contrasting assumptions. In terms of home life, you can make every attempt to expose your child to people and situations that are predictable and within the child's control so that the child learns that she can get herself out of situations when she needs to, is not helpless as she may have felt in the past, and that there are many good and fair people in the world. This exposure to a support network of loving and honorable adults and peers is one of the ingredients for her recovery that Kayla talks about when she contrasts her experiences with the Pedros and the teammates in Boston with what life was like with Daniel.

Themes of reconnecting and reestablishing a healthy self-image and sense of self-determination have been particularly important to Kayla's recovery, and she has more to say about the preceding suggestions in the rest of this chapter.

WATCH FOR ADVANCES IN THE UNDERSTANDING AND TREATMENT OF CSA

As of the publication of this book, complex PTSD is still not a formally recognized diagnosis by the American Psychiatric Association. However, the most recent diagnostic criteria for PTSD now allows for some symptoms that we see in complex PTSD, from dissociation to symptoms in younger children that are distinct from those in adults, such as constricted play and temper tantrums, and negative thoughts and feelings that did not exist before the trauma, including negative core beliefs about oneself and the world and persistent guilt and shame. These revised criteria are an indication of an expanding acceptance, some 40 years after the initial recognition of PTSD as a trauma-induced disorder, of the complex and far-reaching impact of chronic trauma and abuse. This growing acceptance is already leading to advances in treatment, such as the willingness to hasten recovery through inventive ways to allow victims to process the experiences in their past without threatening their present safety. Because recovery can be a long process, it's important to keep up with new developments that may be available to your child or teen in the coming years. Sources of timely information can be found in the Resources.

Kayla is doing her part to advocate for better prevention and intervention by sharing her experiences to increase worldwide awareness of the devastation caused by child sexual abuse. The pervasive impact of her own abuse is reflected clearly in Kayla's journal entry after her McLean admission, when she talks about her ongoing and conflicted preoccupation with Daniel and how his prolonged abuse of her had disrupted, and continued to disrupt, her self-perceptions and core beliefs and distorted her thinking about him:

August 19, 2007 (2 months after being at McLean)

Dear God,

Sometimes I get so sad it hurts. I cry and cry and nobody knows it but me.

I don't remember anything anymore. I don't remember his voice. I can't remember any good times. I only remember times of him screaming at me. I remember Belgium, where he was so proud. I remember being in the car and him screaming at me and calling me a fucking retard.

Sometimes I wonder if it was even real. If he even loved me. And I can't remember. I can't remember how old I really was. Was I 10? 12? And I think back to how I betrayed him. I told our story to everyone and I stabbed him in the back and for that I can never be forgiven.

Love Always,
Kayla

FOSTERING THE NATURAL RECOVERY PROCESS

The outpatient treatment that Kayla was undertaking relied on well-established trauma treatment doctrine dating back to the late 1980s that emphasized the patient's engagement in a therapeutic relationship that *helped the client to first establish safety and then tolerate the reconstruction of the elements of the abuse.* The process of reexposing themselves to trauma-related memories and beliefs in therapy is believed to work for victims at least in part because it replicates the mechanisms of *natural recovery* from trauma. When researchers looked at why some individuals develop PTSD while others do not, they found that sexual abuse survivors who naturally encounter reminders of their trauma during their daily routines, over and over, and keep processing the thoughts and emotions that come up, as well as talking about them, are most likely to process the trauma and recover more fully without the need to do this work in a formal treatment setting. Although Kate Nooner and colleagues have reported in 2012 that while somewhere around 50–60% of teens who experience a known sexual trauma go on to develop clinically significant PTSD, Stephan Collishaw and associates have found evidence that parental and peer support, which may allow for more emotional processing, decreases this likelihood.

| Effective PTSD treatments often mimic the gradual emotional processing that can occur naturally in daily life—but often doesn't without professional help. |

Being able to process the emotions and thoughts that surface in response to trauma is easier with a natural disaster or car accident, because the survivor can talk about it with other people who have witnessed the event. With CSA, the secrecy eliminates this opportunity. This is why psychotherapy can be so helpful to children who have been abused sexually and kept silent about it: it may give them their first chance to reflect and talk about past trauma(s). In this way psychotherapy can reverse one of the main factors that contribute to the development of both PTSD and complex PTSD: the silence that prevents emotional and cognitive processing.

As a parent, you can further your child's recovery not only by making sure she has access to psychotherapy, but also by gently inviting her to talk when you see signs that she is distressed and may be struggling with a reminder of what she went through.

RECONSTRUCTING AND SHARING THE TRAUMA

Many sexually abused children that we've treated have kept some form of private journal, as Kayla did, as one means of coping with their abuse. Journaling provides some opportunity to process the abusive relationship without having to talk with anyone and risk retribution or rejection, but it's typically a mixed blessing, as Kayla realized was the case for her. Kayla's journal provided a critical, private sounding board during the abuse itself, but by allowing her to avoid the shame and confusion she associated with talking to others it kept her silent and limited how much emotional processing she could really do. Fortunately, these journals later helped jog her memory during outpatient therapy about how she had felt and thought at various points in her relationship with Daniel and allowed her to embark on the challenging journey of sharing the details of her past with someone who could now safely bear witness to these distressing past events.

An example of this thought process is seen in one of Kayla's journal entries, where she struggles with whether to let Brian know about her repetitive nightmares of the abuse but assumes that he, like others—like Daniel—would abandon her if she were truthful:

May 28, 2007 (age 16)

Dear God,

   I had the dream again last night. It's hard to differentiate between what's real and what's a dream.
   My mind is like a movie. All the clips keep running through my head. I see him. I see him and I am at his house in his bed. With Jared there and Daniel and I having sex with Jared sleeping in the room.
   And I tell Daniel to stop and I try to get Jared to leave the room. And as I try to leave Daniel grabs me and I wake up in a cold sweat.
   I want to tell someone. I want to tell Brian. If he knew how fucked up I was I'm sure he'd run as fast as far away as he could.
   If he could hear my screams or see my thoughts he'd run.
   Sometimes I just want him to know so bad but just when I'm about to open my mouth and let my soul pour out I realize that I can never again trust someone the way I trusted Daniel.
   But I want to.

   Love Always,
   Kayla

Another way that journaling became a springboard for Kayla's recovery efforts was in reconstructing her narrative in writing. Along with verbally relating one's trauma story, a written reconstruction has been found to be one of the most effective strategies for dealing with trauma-related distress. In fact it's incorporated as a formal element in several of the evidence-based treatments reviewed in Chapter 6. Reconstructing a traumatic experience in therapy, either spoken or written, and outside of therapy when ready, has been shown to help trauma victims organize the memories and feelings into a more manageable and understandable psychological package. Some of the exposure-based treatments in wide use today, in fact, rely on the prolonged or repeated retelling that often begins with writing the details of a traumatic event to achieve optimal results. Edna Foa, the

treatment originator of prolonged exposure (see Chapter 6), and colleagues state in their 2008 book that repeated talking and thinking
about a memory via imaginal exposure helps traumatized individuals:

- Organize the memory.
- Get used to the fear and/or anxiety associated with the mem-
  ory.
- Resist the urge to avoid the memories and triggers of them.

How does this work? The reconstruction can rely on original writings, reflections in hindsight, or accounts of others that corroborate
what happened. It typically takes place gradually, over an extended
period of time. Most victims of sexual trauma say it's the narrative
process itself, rather than the production of a finished story, that
feels most therapeutic. *They often talk about experiencing a sense of profound mastery at being finally able to put into words what originally happened
to them under a shroud of silence and secrecy.* And that sense of control
over events that at one point felt overwhelmingly out of their control
increases at every stage of telling. Reconstructing and sharing these
experiences diminish distress and confusion, and as time goes on the
details become less overwhelming. Victims describe at some point in
this process feeling that they are finally moving from *victim* to *survivor*.
As Ellen Bass and Laura Davis described it almost 40 years ago in their
now iconic book *The Courage to Heal,*

> It is possible to heal. It is even possible to thrive. Thriving means
> more than just an alleviation of symptoms, more than Band-Aids,
> more than functioning adequately. Thriving means enjoying a feel-
> ing of wholeness, satisfaction in your life and work, genuine love
> and trust in your relationships, pleasure in your body. . . . So often
> survivors have had their experiences denied, trivialized, or dis-
> torted. Writing is an important avenue for healing because it gives
> you the opportunity to define your own reality. You can say: This
> did happen to me. It was that bad. It was the fault & responsibility
> of the adult. I was—and am—innocent.

As parents, we may not ever get to see or hear the reconstruction
of the trauma, and that is often as it should be. Some children need an
objective, trained adult to help them reveal and then organize what
they went through in their abuse, and these details remain too

difficult to share with family members. Often all a parent can either know or ask about is what progress the child is making in sharing and processing past events and has to rely on the child's behaviors as the indicator of whether she is recovering. For example, is the child less isolated, less angry, and more interactive at home?

> Victims benefit from writing about and telling their stories in a multitude of ways, and it is essential that we all stand ready to listen.

RECONNECTING

Trusting, close connections with others are important to everyone's well-being, and they are particularly vital to victims of child sexual abuse. But it can obviously be a challenge to reestablish such relationships when you've learned through a harrowing pattern of abuse that those who are supposed to protect you can't be trusted. Generally speaking, as their trauma reactions and current triggers are better understood, child and teen survivors often find they can manage symptoms better and have fewer urges to engage in unhelpful and risky behaviors. The combination of insights gained about the trauma and the trust developed within a therapeutic relationship also tends to reduce withdrawal and isolation and help the victims reestablish first trust and then intimacy with people in their lives.

This gradual process of reconnecting began to unfold for Kayla outside of therapy during the years between her admission to McLean and the climb toward her first Olympics, as she was finally able to explore being in a close relationship again:

Relearning how to love someone can be a hard thing. I'm not necessarily talking about other people, but about myself. For a very long time I did not love myself. I felt dirty, used, and broken. I felt like I was damaged goods—how could anyone ever love me? Because of this mentality, reconnecting with people on an intimate level was a big challenge. Both physically and emotionally.

I was engaged to be married right before the Olympics in London. On the outside everything seemed perfect. And even in the relationship I fooled myself into thinking it was okay. I thought it was okay if I didn't want to have sex but I faked it. I thought it was okay to cry sometimes after and feel an emptiness inside. My partner was the most patient, understanding man, but for a long, long time

I wasn't patient with myself. I didn't listen to myself. I struggled to be the girl I thought I should be versus just being me. And this ultimately caused too much damage to sustain our relationship.

Looking back, I wish I had been honest. With myself and with him. I wasn't ready for a lot of it. I couldn't handle a lot of it, but I tried to power through and get to somewhere I wasn't ready to be. This is one of the hardest things to overcome, in my opinion, after being sexually abused.

You have to stop trying to please everyone and listen to yourself. You have to know your triggers and realize it takes time to overcome them. You have to be patient with yourself. And learning to be intimate again is one thing you cannot power through. It takes time, patience, and unconditional love for yourself. You are not perfect. You are not always going to be happy. You are not always going to feel empowered or smart or beautiful or strong or brave. But you have to give yourself time to become all of those things. You can never learn to trust another in the most intimate way if you never learn to trust yourself again.

Over the years I have had several boyfriends and close relationships. And anytime things seem to be going wrong I find myself thinking it's me. I find myself wondering if there's something wrong with me. I wonder if I'm just too messed up to be loved. I still find myself having these thoughts, to this day. But sex has equaled love to me for a long time. It's meant that everything's okay. And I'm only just now, at 27, learning that sex doesn't mean love. It is an important part for sure, and it is something every relationship needs, but it isn't the sum total of a partnership. It's okay to say no. That is the hardest lesson I have had to learn in my journey to healing. Not just in love but in life. It's okay to not do everything for everyone all the time. It's okay to just think of yourself.

If you want to love someone, you have to learn to love all of you. The bad parts, the worst parts of you. The dirty secrets and the sad ones. The highs and the lows. You have to love yourself unconditionally. And it's a lesson I'm still learning.

Depending on who the perpetrator was and what his relationship was to the victim's family and friends, it can also take some time before an abused child feels comfortable in relationships with relatives and peers. In instances where the perpetrator is an adult who also has relationships with the child's peers and/or relatives, as in the cases of a coach, teacher, or clergy member, it's equally important to be able to approach, rather than avoid, a discussion of the reality of the abuse. Kayla found herself wary of those in the judo community in Ohio because they all knew about Daniel's abuse of her, and unkind rumors and speculation had been circulated in the press. She also at times found her relationship with her immediate family challenged by her anger at her parents for not recognizing that Daniel was abusing her, even though he had practically become a member of the family and had worked hard to gain their trust:

> While writing this book I have encountered many tough questions about myself and my life. Some so deep and buried I've had to write and then cry and write and then cry and write and then scream. It's not easy talking about the past, but I've found it's even harder talking about the present. Some areas I have fooled myself into thinking were okay but they weren't.
>
> I have been angry with my mother for a very, very long time. I have been angry since I was 16. I have also loved my mother, and she has tried to love me through it all. Though I didn't always make it easy for her.
>
> When I first moved to Boston, I would go months without seeing her, or speaking to her. I would ignore every phone call and the ones I would take would usually end with me screaming into the phone. Then came the period where a very tense and fragile truce was made. I turned 18. I wasn't a child anymore (even though it felt as if I hadn't been one for years). I was in control of my life, and so I let go of a little bit of anger. But I always made it hard for my mom. I kept her at arm's distance. I let her know I was okay without her. I had grown up. I could do this on my own. I didn't need her. I pushed her away all the while loving her and hating her.
>
> While writing this book the one person I wanted to protect wasn't myself; it was my mom. I didn't want her to know how angry I was and how little I had done to fix it. I didn't want her to be judged on her decisions because I know and she knows she did the best that she could. Talking to her about what happened has helped us heal a lot. But we're still not perfect. I still find a small glimmer of that anger of a 16-year-old left to herself and judo burning inside. It's been 10 years and I still feel it. I don't know that it will ever

FIGHTING BACK

go away. But I know for sure it won't if I don't try. I know for sure nothing will change if I refuse to talk and open up and be honest. Not just with her but with myself.

Is my anger misdirected sometimes? Absolutely. I get angry at my mom for calling Daniel a monster. Why? Of course she feels that way—she's my mother and he hurt me in the most intimate way a human can hurt a child. He stole my innocence, and yet I feel anger at her. I get angry over silly things like her need to try to make the best of every situation. I find it exhausting to try to pretend, and I refuse a lot of times to go along with it and smile when I don't want to. I smile for the rest of the world, so why should I have to smile for her? I think all the time. I use my past as a crutch to not try to see a better future between us, and the result for our relationship is not just her fault, it's mine.

It takes a long time to heal. It's a long long journey. And being honest with yourself and the ones closest to you is the only way to take a step forward. I hope my mother knows I'm trying. I hope she reads this book and feels my love for her more than my anger. I hope she knows that I know she did the right things. I hope she knows that it wasn't her fault. And because of her strength, I was able to begin to heal. And because of her strength, hopefully many more people will take that first step on the path to healing.

Incest, of course, is particularly difficult. It can take an extended time period for family members to interact constructively with one another, as there is often anger and guilt and a great deal of confusion about the incestuous relationship. In this situation it is important to try to talk as openly as possible about the abuse, so that the natural recovery process can help family members understand and accept what transpired. It is through this interpersonal engagement that trust is restored and the child can once again feel reconnected rather than isolated. Additionally, incest can be challenging in that it often ends in the disconnection of the entire family from the identified perpetrator, be that a sibling, father, or other close relative. Individual family members can find it difficult to provide continued support to the victim when they might still either disbelieve the accusation in some measure or, alternatively, be so angry with the perpetrator that their feelings prevent their maintaining a compassionate stance toward the individual who has been abused. As we discussed earlier, an abuse victim (and this can be especially true in cases of incest) can have an array of both positive and negative feelings toward the abuser following disclosure, and the anger and vengeful reactions of others can then hinder the processing of the trauma and the victim's recovery.

In cases of incest, it's wise to ensure that all family members have a chance to talk with a trained professional about their reactions and to seek advice about how to mutually support one another. If you or the child's other parent feels so responsible for and unresolved about the sexual abuse—say when it is your husband or father who was the perpetrator—it might also be wise to seek your own personal treatment. Children are typically very sensitive to how people in the family are coping following an incest disclosure, and they need to see that others can "handle the truth" and that their further processing is not met with escalating distress and crisis.

A Message for Parents

Looking back, it's easy for me to make suggestions on what parents can do to try to help their child through this difficult time. But I am not a parent. I have never felt the overwhelming sensation of love for a child. So I cannot imagine what hurt and anger and feeling of failure comes with the thought of having not seen the abuse or been able to stop it.

I think the biggest thing a parent can do to try to help the healing process is compassion. I know you are suffering, but so is your child. Rage and revenge can fuel you, but you should not let your child see that. You must be strong for the child and at times demand she get professional help or urge her to cooperate with the authorities, but you must balance that with a compassion and an understanding that your child is wounded. Your child now has deep, deep wounds even if they are not visible to the human eye. And it's going to take a long time and a lot of work to heal those wounds. It's been 10 years, and I'm still constantly working on it, as well as my mother.

I suggest family counseling. Let your child talk to you, and if it's too hard, bring in someone else to help guide those conversations. Be willing to listen and really hear your child. He may have felt love for his abuser, he may have hated him. I can assure that no matter what the circumstance is your child is feeling a deep guilt and probable self-loathing. The child will probably be angry with the world. He will probably want to shut down. Support him. Let him know you are there for him and you love him no matter what. Seek professional help to allow your child to develop coping skills and tools to go out in the world and deal with this abuse. And always, always, always show strength in this time of adversity. Be the example and let your child know that it's going to be okay. You will get through this, together.

BUILDING MASTERY AND RECOVERY

Developing an understanding and acceptance of the past is only part of the recovery process. It needs to be reinforced with opportunities for establishing mastery and control in ongoing everyday life. Survivors and scholars alike consistently point to finding a way to live one's life with meaning and a sense of value as a necessary antidote to the aftereffects of suffering sexual abuse. For Kayla the route to feeling a sense of mastery and control was her athletic prowess and promise. When she realized through insights gained in therapy that she could still be special, even one-of-a-kind, without having to endure violations and deceptions, she was able to fully reengage in judo training and competition. As a result she won meet after meet and became physically stronger every day. In turn, her tournament medals came to symbolize much more than her athletic prowess—a deep psychological transcendence from sexual abuse victim to survivor.

Establishing areas of excellence that can help a child feel in control and competent is considered a key component in recovery from childhood abuse. An extensive literature has examined the components of what is termed *resiliency,* or the capacity to endure and transcend severe life stressors. What is generally found is that while some aspects of resiliency may be inherited or biological, other aspects have to do with an individual's ability and willingness to reconnect with a positive social and community network, as well as having an opportunity for competent functioning in an area tied to the individual's personal goals.

The Role of Self-Efficacy in Recovery

The harrowing experience of sexual abuse, particularly in childhood and adolescence, is associated with lower self-efficacy, defined as the belief in one's own ability to effectively exercise control and function competently within a given situation, as reported by Britain

Lamoureaux and colleagues in 2012. Self-efficacy is often impaired in these children, taking shape as significant decreases in self-esteem, mastery, and agency following the abuse. In the past a lot of attention was paid to the ways that this loss of self-efficacy can result in more sustained negative outcomes, but more attention has been given recently to how *improving* self-efficacy might influence important steps in the recovery process.

At its core, self-efficacy rests on self-esteem. Self-esteem is based on a person's belief that she can succeed in reaching goals, based on her past experience. Obviously then, having opportunities to *set and achieve goals through her own actions and preparation* can strengthen someone's self-esteem and self-efficacy.

This, in essence, is why "strength-based wellness counseling" has become important. In this more concrete, forward-looking therapeutic approach, children who have been sexually abused are assisted in setting and reaching goals for which they are highly motivated and that require full engagement with a specific task. This approach is showing promise in helping survivors learn to persist despite challenges, increase their willingness to ask for and accept help from others to achieve their goals, and develop renewed confidence in their capacity for success. And it is these very principles, imparted to her by the Pedros, that Kayla believes promoted her psychological healing as much as traditional therapy.

While recognizing that not every child has the athletic potential to become an Olympic champion, it is Kayla's firm belief that every child can, and needs to, set goals for herself that are just out of reach and then engage in a mentored journey to reach those goals. It matters not whether these goals are athletic, academic, or artistic, or about making a particular contribution to others; what matters is that victims can develop confidence that they have survived and can continue to survive in spite of sometimes difficult odds—that they can feel a sense of accomplishment rather than helplessness.

I think one key thing is having something to focus on, having a goal. And that's what I talk about during my speeches. I say that it doesn't have to be an Olympic gold medal. Whatever your goal is, you need to wake up every day and you need to have a purpose. I sat down with Jimmy at the beginning of every year, and I would write down goals. I would write down three goals inside of judo and three goals outside of judo and then key areas that I needed to focus on in order to reach those goals. Maybe someday someone's goal is to be a doctor, but if you're 16, that's a long way away. So my goal was to be an Olympic champion, but when I was 16 my goal was to be national champion or top 10 in the world or to get my black belt. It's something that you can literally focus on every day, and that's what I tell people all the time. There are always baby steps. That's what I tell them. It wasn't like one day I just woke up and I was all better. Baby steps, it was one foot in front of the other. And it was little tiny, tiny wins.

What was super important to me, and what's something I still think about every day, is I train my mind the same way I train my body. I use positive thinking and visualization and I use those to be successful or I go to therapy because I think it's important to have a healthy mind and be able to talk to someone and to be able to figure out what coping skills you need and what you need to work on. I said my mind is just as important for what I do as my body is, so for instance, when I had reconstructive knee surgery, every night I would visualize my knee getting better. I would visualize things starting to work again. Before the Olympics every night before I went to bed I would visualize a perfect day at the Olympics. I would visualize winning the Olympics over and over and over again. Whatever it is, you have to mentally believe it.

FINDING—AND MAKING—MEANING

For Kayla judo was both her passion and at times her nemesis, and the conviction and support of others kept her going when she temporarily lost faith. Kayla appreciates that having a goal and getting support in achieving it was fundamental to her personal triumph. With her continued commitment to writing, sparring, and retelling her personal story in therapy, Kayla eventually arrived at a fuller appreciation that her early abuse was indeed over. With this realization came a renewed determination to reach her childhood dream, once derailed, of being an Olympian. By 2010 Kayla had won the World Judo Championship after competing and medaling in numerous other national and international tournaments. By 2011, as Kayla prepared for the London Olympics, her fame as a potential U.S. medal contender in judo had made her an increasingly public figure and someone the sports press was interested in interviewing. Then that fall, before the

London games, while Kayla trained rigorously with the Pedros and Daniel remained behind bars serving a sentence of 10 years in prison without the possibility of parole, Kayla again began to think of all the other children and teens who she now realized were also victims of CSA, many of whom still lived in their own prisons fashioned from silence and shame:

> While training for the London Olympics the Jerry Sandusky case was coming to light. And in the light of that, while I had not spoken publicly, I felt compelled to do so. The night before the first article was to be published I got in a heated debate with one of my friends regarding the Jerry Sandusky scandal and the ultimate firing of Joe Paterno. My friend has posted that JoPa didn't deserve to be fired, and I remember seeing on the news Penn State students rioting and flipping over cars because of this. And I couldn't believe that I lived in a world where students and my peers were rioting over a football coach losing his job, but not rioting for the countless victims whose lives had forever been changed by one man's actions. And I realized in that moment it was because they didn't understand. They couldn't see the victims. They didn't realize it was their friends, their peers. They didn't have a face or a voice. And so I decided to be that face. I decided to be that voice. And from that day on I made a decision to never be silent again.

Although most people in the judo community realized from the time of Daniel's arrest and sentencing that Kayla had been his victim, she herself had never been publicly identified, but named only by initials (KH) in court documents. It would have stayed that way had Kayla not chosen to redirect the spotlight shined on her by the Olympics toward the very personal goal of helping raise awareness about the horrors of child sexual abuse. Recognizing that many victims were struggling to recover without the benefit of the supportive family, Olympic-level talent, or access to the top-notch psychiatric care that she had, Kayla decided she might be able to prevent some children from being the victims of this enduring danger:

> After deciding to speak out, I slowly became much more involved with the system and the many victims of CSA. And I realized we have a long way to go in terms of helping with the aftermath of abuse. One key thing for me is education. In health class as a young

adolescent I learned about stranger danger. I learned about saying no to drugs. I learned safe sex practices and what you should do when being peer pressured. But I never learned what you should do if someone close to you or an adult in power tries to take advantage of you. I never learned what grooming was. I never learned it's okay to say no to an adult. Or to tell someone if someone close does try to do any of those things. And that, to me, is a major flaw in our quest to stamp out sexual abuse. Knowledge and education is power. It is a way we can empower our children and let them know how to deal with the possibility of sexual abuse. I'm not suggesting everyone will be abused or that we should sleep with one eye open, but we should know the signs. We should be aware. We should take caution. If you have a child, I urge you to share what you've learned in this book with them. I urge you to take steps and begin to have the conversation.

Sexual abuse thrives in the silence. This book is a tool and a way to never let that silence grow so loud that we can't hear our children. It is a way to fight back.

Perhaps, Kayla thought, her story could help thousands of young people still too confused and afraid to speak up about their sexual abuse. Maybe she could give parents and caretakers valuable information about what to look for and how to intervene. Based on this conviction, Kayla made what was likely the bravest decision of her life. She chose to break her silence once more and go public with the account of her abuse, first in an interview that ran in *USA Today* in 2011 and then in a feature article in *Sports Illustrated* in December 2012, after she won the Olympic Gold medal in London. Kayla has not stopped speaking out since then, using her public engagements and media presence to add her voice to efforts focused on raising awareness and providing education concerning the risks and prevention of child sexual abuse (see Chapter 8).

In the now famous *Sports Illustrated* article, "Stand Up and Speak Out," Kayla talks of how she yearned as a child for someone to figure out what was going on and *rescue* her. The fact that Kayla now realizes she suffered long after the abuse, not just during it, fueled her determination to use her personal story as part of a larger mission to ensure that victimized children get the help they so desperately need in a timely manner. Although no one came to Kayla's rescue during the time she was abused, because no one had the necessary knowledge to do so, Kayla is grateful that her mother, coaches, and peers paid close attention to her distress following disclosure and once she was in treatment and did all the right things:

- Finding professional treatment when Kayla became unsafe and troubled in a way they could not manage.
- Insisting that she go for ongoing counseling.
- Supporting her gradual efforts to talk, reconnect, and trust others again.
- Providing her with opportunities to return to an activity she loved and excelled at—judo.
- Insisting that Kayla learn to be self-sufficient and disciplined, which, in turn, restored her sense of self-esteem and mastery.

If the adults in Kayla's life had known more about the *how* and *who* of child sexual abuse, Kayla might have been spared years of suffering—suffering that at times almost cost Kayla her life. At that time, however, little was known not only about how to identify child sexual abuse but also about the process of recovery and what therapeutic and practical interventions are most effective in this effort. Fortunately, educational efforts have made strides toward preventing other children and teens from meeting the same fate and in disseminating important information about how to help victims make their way back to living a full and meaningful life.

8

How We Can All Help

PREVENTION AND EDUCATION

> My judo legacy is fulfilled, and I'm happy . . . I'm happy
> with my career. Now it's time to go and continue to add
> to the legacy off the mat and try and change the world.
> —Kayla's first comments following her gold medal win,
>   Rio Olympic Games, 2016

Following her gold medal triumph in London in 2012, Kayla continued to speak out publicly and share her personal story as a means
of alerting others to the dangers of child sexual abuse. Her pioneering interviews in *USA Today* and *Sports Illustrated* were met with an
outcry of appreciation that Kayla had not anticipated, as fellow victims and their parents reached out to express their gratitude. Kayla's
speaking up, they said, had helped many others step forward as well
and brought to the forefront the need for more awareness and prevention education. Almost everyone, whether emailing or stopping Kayla
on her way to catch a plane, said, "This happened to me, and I can't
believe it happened to you too . . . how can we make this stop?"

The response spurred Kayla to use the media spotlight she had
as a Gold Medal Olympian to address audiences whenever and wherever she could to raise public awareness about this important public health issue. In an interview with ESPNW's Allison Glock in July
2016, before she defended her gold medal in the Rio Olympics, Kayla
talked in detail about the impact of her abuse and the toll she knew
that being victimized had on other victims.

You can't physically see that I'm wounded, . . . but when you're 10 or 12 years old, and you go through something like that, it . . . leaves scars all over your heart . . .

One time after I shared my story, this girl walked up to me and handed me a note, and she said, "Just read it later . . ." That night I was on the plane and I pulled out the note. It said: "Kayla, I was raped a month ago. And it's really hard for me to get out of bed. But you give me hope that someday I will. Thank you." That was so powerful to me, that my speaking out or sharing my story can affect someone that much and give them hope. To me, that's bigger and better than any gold medal will ever be.

This excerpt, from one of Kayla's many media interviews in 2016, captures the fervor of what had become a 4-year personal mission for Kayla after winning her first gold medal. It was also after that victory that Kayla had contacted one of us, Dr. Kaplan, whom she knew from her time at McLean, to discuss how she might most effectively use her personal story of recovery and now highly celebrated status to increase public awareness of child sexual abuse. The idea of using Kayla's writings, both those from her childhood journal and the later recollections that formed the basis of her reconstructed trauma narrative, as a vehicle to reach a larger and more sustained audience than was possible through individual interviews and articles began to take shape, but this book had to be set aside while Kayla focused on defending her gold medal title in Rio in 2016.

Then, literally in the immediate aftermath of her gold medal win, as the furor in Rio subsided, Kayla responded to one of her many congratulatory emails from her fans in Boston and at McLean Hospital:

On September 7, 2016, at 9:47 A.M.

Dr. Kaplan!

Thank you so so much!

I am so glad you emailed! I have been sitting here pretty much every day since I won thinking about how to start an email to you and what to say and here buried in all of my emails is one from you!

I know it has been a long time, and I know I sort of just went off the grid, but if you are willing and able still—I am ready to write that book. I have lots of responsibilities but I am no longer training, so my days are very long and I am looking forward to doing what I set out to do all those months ago with you.

I am in Ohio for a celebration but will be in town next week. I would love to come to your office to meet and discuss if it helps. Or even just take you to lunch somewhere.

I understand if things for you have changed or if you are no longer able to work with me and realize I could not really focus my attention and time on this project while I was training and competing. I won't be at all offended if you are no longer interested. But since you emailed and since it is still a dream of mine I thought it couldn't hurt to ask.

I hope you are well and I look forward to hearing from you.

Best,
Kayla

With this email, Kayla and her writing team returned to the idea of using Kayla's personal story as a cautionary tale to help others. Kayla had never stopped using writing to come to terms with what she had gone through, and she continued to consider ways in which this personal narrative might be useful to other survivors, as well as to prevent child sexual abuse from happening at all.

The revelation of what had happened to her daughter shattered Kayla's mother, Jeannie Yazell, whose worries about Daniel had been initially dispelled by Kayla's refutations along with her own lack of knowledge about sexual abuse of children. She had never heard of *grooming*, and had no idea about the frequency with which coaches and adults in positions of power abuse children in their care. "Our society," says Yazell, "definitely didn't educate me on what to look for. I could never imagine or believe someone close to us could take advantage of my child. They don't talk about that in nursing school, they don't talk about that in the school system. I don't know if I was in denial, but I could never imagine this was happening to Kayla."

It was in this context that we sought to learn as much as we could about the approaches others had taken to increasing public awareness and providing necessary education, education about preventing sexual abuse that Kayla and her mother unfortunately never had the benefit of at the time when the abuse began. Kayla's mother believes that if she had only had more information at the time, more facts, she might have been able to intervene and spare her daughter years of emotional damage and trauma. So as this book started to take shape, we devoted considerable time to reviewing what had been tried, and what had worked, in initiatives designed to tackle the prevention and awareness of sexual abuse in childhood.

Delphine Collin-Vézina and associates of McGill University emphasized in 2013 that there is no doubt that child sexual abuse is a health epidemic of major proportions and that efforts and resources need to be aimed at prevention education. Although a majority of victims never report their abuse during childhood, according to the latest accounting from the National Child Abuse and Neglect Data System (NCANDS) report of 2016, there were over 58,000 substantiated cases of child sexual abuse in the United States for the year 2014 (*www.acf.hhs.gov/cb/resource/child-maltreatment-2014*). Given the extent of this wide-ranging problem, over the past several decades a considerable range of efforts have been undertaken to increase awareness and promote prevention. Some of them are mandated by law; some have been spearheaded by the private sector. Some are focused on managing perpetrators and potential perpetrators, and others are focused on the victims or potential victims. Programs are delivered either through the schools or in the community. All are aimed at reducing the incidence and toll of this epidemic, and they have experienced varying success.

Our research was originally intended to help Kayla determine where and how to best focus her own efforts to boost awareness and promote education, but you can use the following information to find programs in your own community, whether to enhance your own understanding of the problem, to get involved in advocacy efforts, or to help initiatives reach the many innocent children and teens who deserve to be protected. We hope that reading about these efforts will give you a greater awareness of child maltreatment and reassure you that you are not alone if someone you care about has been victimized.

OFFENDER-MANAGEMENT
VERSUS VICTIM-FOCUSED INITIATIVES

For the last several decades one of the major initiatives for preventing the sexual victimization of children has involved what is termed *offender management,* focusing resources on controlling the whereabouts of known or suspected perpetrators and employing tactics that include setting up registry systems for convicted offenders, community notification programs, implementing background check requirements for employment, and efforts to control the charging, sentencing, and parole parameters for convicted offenders.

In general, these offender-centered initiatives have not been rigorously evaluated, and their major shortcoming resides in the reality that they can only directly affect those perpetrators who have already been adjudicated, leaving many potential offenders at large and unsupervised. In terms of Kayla's personal experience, she was heartened to learn that her former coach would be supervised once released from prison to minimize the likelihood that he could reoffend, and that he was also banned for life from working as a judo coach, thus reducing the potential opportunities for Daniel, like many other coaches, educators, and clergy in the past, to use their position and power to again gain access to a vulnerable child or teen.

In our estimation, however, efforts that stress awareness and monitoring of offenders' penalties and whereabouts, over prevention and timely detection, have some serious drawbacks. Specifically, Kayla was intent on finding out about, and contributing to, initiatives that were geared toward facilitating the earlier discovery and disclosure of sexually abusive relationships during childhood, thus potentially interrupting relationships like the one she had endured from age 12 to 16. David Finkelhor, a pioneer in the field, echoes Kayla's reservation about offender programs in his observation that "only a small percentage of new offenders have a prior sex offense record that would have involved them in the management system" and recommends using societal resources to identify the "concealed" offenders who pose the greatest threat to children and concentrate comprehensive management efforts only on those at the highest risk of reoffending.

Historically it's been the tragic individual experiences of particular victims and their families that have led to increased advocacy and the enactment of legislative changes critical to preventing abuse. In the past decade, high-profile sexual abuse scandals involving clergy and educational and youth organization staff (such as in the Jerry Sandusky case) have resulted in greater public awareness of the nature and scale of this phenomenon, a problem the American Medical Association aptly described in 1995 as "a silent, violent epidemic." This awareness has led to an increase in advocacy spearheaded by foundations and other organizations in the private sector. As an example, Joe Paterno's widow, Sue Paterno, and other family members began collaborating with Stop It Now!, an organization initially established by Fran Henry, herself a sexual abuse survivor, and have worked collaboratively to develop the Circles of Safety for Higher Education program to combat child sexual victimization by working with university systems to train staff in child sexual abuse prevention. The idea here is for university systems, which are often used as settings for activities and camps for minor children, to set new guidelines for protecting youth by training college staff members to recognize the warning signs of child sexual abuse. In addition to the Paternos' foundation, many other such organizations have been formed to help combat child sexual abuse, including:

- the NoVo Foundation, which donated a total of $5 million between 2009 and 2012 to the Ms. Foundation for Women to support a project called Child Sexual Abuse: A Social Justice Prevention Model.

- the Robert Wood Johnson Foundation, which donated $500,000 in 2011 to the Chicago Children's Advocacy Center to "support the Network of Treatment Providers Collaborative Project in expanding mental health treatment for victims of child sexual abuse."

- the OAK Foundation, which donates millions of dollars annually, both nationally and internationally, to support initiatives that eliminate the sexual exploitation of children, engage men and boys in combating the sexual abuse of children, and promote the prevention of violence against children.

Wider publicity has also resulted in legislation designed to increase awareness and education to prevent child sexual abuse, and it's gratifying to see that a majority of states have signed up for some form of legislated protection. As of August 2015, only 26 states and the territory of Guam were at various stages of implementing some type of legislative mandate for states to address the need to prevent CSA, and many of these legislative mandates did no more than direct states to form task forces to examine the issue; they don't legislate any specific actions. In comparison, 31 states by this time in 2017 are *requiring* school districts (as part of what is generally referred to as Erin's Law, discussed shortly, to provide a prevention-oriented curriculum for students, school personnel, and parents to promote "awareness and prevention training on child sexual abuse," within 1 year of passage). To see what legislation has been enacted in your state, check the website of the National Conference for State Legislatures (*https:// tinyurl.com/m4nme8v*).

Although initially designed and then mandated for school delivery, sexual abuse prevention programs have also more recently been successfully integrated into various education programs within religious institutions and other youth-focused organizations (e.g., Boys and Girls Clubs), and the last several decades have seen an increase in the number of nonprofit organizations dedicated to increasing community awareness and prevention. Campaigns that have most recently been waged to raise CSA awareness and in the process boost prevention without being required by law are many and varied, ranging from the designation of April as Sexual Assault Awareness Month (SAAM) in the United States (*www.nsvrc.org/saam*), as part of a campaign originally started by the Pennsylvania Coalition Against Rape, to White Balloon Day, which is Australia's largest and longest-running child protection campaign, now in its 21st year, dedicated to the prevention of child sexual assault and encouragement for victims to break their silence by speaking out.

Whether child sexual abuse is combated through legislation or initiatives instigated privately, there is no doubt of the powerful impact victims can have, and have had, on child awareness and protection policy, legislation, and program implementation and delivery. For example, Erin's Law, first passed in Illinois in 2011, is a state law requiring school-based education for CSA prevention. Named after an adult survivor, Erin Merryn, who suffered years of sexual assault by an uncle as a young child and then later was victimized by an older cousin, the law mandates that public schools develop age-appropriate materials to teach students in grades K–12 how to come forward if they are being sexually abused and to instruct staff on how to handle such revelations. Erin disclosed her abuse to local authorities at age 13. With the goal of using her own experience to prevent other children from suffering as she had, Erin successfully advocated that other states pass similar laws. As of the writing of this book 31 states have enacted some version of Erin's law requiring schools to begin to either "study or develop age-appropriate child sexual abuse identification and prevention curricula for pre-K through the 5th, 8th, or 12th grade to help children, teachers, and parents recognize and identify child sexual abuse" and to implement these programs either immediately or following a restricted, year-long period for development prior to implementation (National Conference of State Legislatures, Child Sexual Prevention: Erin's Law, 2015). And Erin is far from the only survivor who has left her mark. Jenna Quinn, a sexual abuse survivor, engineered Jenna's Law, which mandates that all public schools, charter schools, and day care facilities train staff and parents on the signs and symptoms of all forms of child abuse in Texas. Kat Alexander, an incest survivor, is the 35-year-old founder and CEO of *Report It, Girl,* a website for and by survivors that aims to foster healing, awareness, and community through attaching language to experience— expressive writing about trauma—to promote healing. These survivors, along with many others, have turned their personal experiences into a mission to help other child sexual abuse victims.

As a fellow survivor, Kayla had the opportunity to get to know Erin Merryn personally and lend her own voice to the important challenge of influencing public health policy and legislation in the area of CSA prevention and awareness education. Kayla has also devoted her time to working with countless private and public organizations in an effort to make a difference in the lives of victims of childhood sexual abuse via advocacy for legislative change.

Our society abhors the victimization of children through sexual abuse, and the massive publicity around horrific stories, such as that of Jerry Sandusky at Penn State University and those of the priests in Boston, have resulted in major prevention efforts. The Stop It Now! Foundation, noted earlier, disseminates knowledge about recognizing and preventing CSA by training education professionals. We've also seen Boston's Catholic schools adopt the Committee for Children's Talking About Touching program, a pre-K–3 program taught in 25,000 schools nationwide, after revelations of widespread abuse there brought the problem to the Church's attention.

We encourage you to consider getting involved too. Many adults who care about a child who has been victimized feel empowered by helping with advocacy efforts. See the Resources for information on organizations that can help you get involved in supporting advocacy against sexual abuse and in ensuring that awareness and prevention continue to be a focus of policymakers and all those charged with protecting our youth. Also be sure to find out what kinds of educational and prevention programs are available in your community.

SCHOOL-BASED EDUCATIONAL PROGRAMS

As described earlier, a small majority of states have enacted legislation requiring that schools develop educational curricula designed to prevent, and not only identify and report, child sexual abuse. These programs teach children skills such as how to recognize unsafe situations and relationships, identify grooming behaviors, separate from uncomfortable interactions, and seek appropriate help when necessary. They also aim to encourage disclosure, and many teach principles of bystander intervention. Where there is legislative support for these efforts, instructive material on child sexual abuse has been integrated into a broader school-based mental health and safety promotion curriculum. Public schools have the decided advantage in disseminating this information as educators have access to nearly all children and their families during the primary and secondary school years; in many states schools have readily accepted responsibility for this educational task.

Thus far, the evidence we have suggests that school-based awareness programs are an effective method for addressing a variety of prevention goals, including teaching refusal skills to children and teens, providing deterrence messages to potential adolescent offenders, and promoting assistance skills for bystanders. By many estimates a third of offenders are juveniles themselves, although they are over the age of consent with a victim who is under the age of consent. These programs are intended not only to teach girls to say no but also to educate boys who would potentially offend to think again and to intervene and/or say something if they witness an incident involving one of their peers.

The same approaches used in these school-based programs can be encouraged at home, as home is where children first learn about how people in society are expected to behave. Changing social norms that accept or allow indifference to sexual abuse is one of the goals for school-based programs. Being taught to be acquiescent can be a problem for girls who are touched inappropriately. Encouraging aggression and promoting the idea of sexual contact as a means of conquest can be a problem for boys trying to learn social norms of behavior around girls and women. These are the societal messages that need to change, and these changes can be encouraged by parents:

• *Change Male Norms:* Work with your child to make sure that you are fostering healthy, positive norms about masculinity, gender, and violence, particularly for young boys. It means paying attention to the messages about sexual violence in the media and supervising the content they are exposed to at a young age. Model respectful behavior toward women within the household and consider ways at home to demonstrate that "no means no" where touching of any kind is concerned and that boys and men must act as allies, not antagonists, to girls and women.

- *Empower Girls:* This approach reinforces the message that girls have power in relationships by recognizing the emotional and physical barriers that often inhibit actions in female children and by helping your daughter to assert herself in situations where the prevailing sex role norms might include acquiescing to boys or men because of societal expectations and differences in strength and physical size. It involves learning to identify situations early on where they are beginning to feel coerced, uncomfortable, or bullied and to use verbal and physical strategies to refuse contact, find ways to escape the situation, and, most important, feel comfortable telling you or another safe adult what is happening!

- *Teach Bystander Awareness:* This is important for male and female children alike and really is about directly teaching your children to intervene if someone they know is being hurt—it comes down to the adage "see something . . . do something." It involves talking to them at home about the importance of peer leadership and how their observations and actions can help prevent someone else from being hurt. Part of this means helping them in everyday situations to see behaviors—aggressiveness as a means of getting what you want, misogynistic talk, for instance—that potentially put others at risk of being victimized and taking appropriate steps to intervene effectively, whether directly or by promptly enlisting the help of an adult.

To date studies that specifically examined the success of a variety of school-based CSA awareness and prevention programs have yielded encouraging, if not conclusive, findings. One such study by Gibson and Leitenberg in 2000 asked 825 college students about their participation, as children, in a school-based prevention program that included a focus on CSA. These authors found that young women who had prior awareness and prevention education were only about half as likely to have been sexually abused as children as their peers without the same educational exposure. Another study, however, reviewed by David Finkelhor in 2009 looked at youth ages 10–16 and found no significant difference in the rate of victimization when comparing those who had and had not participated in a comprehensive prevention program. Program participation was, however, associated with a personal sense of mastery in the handling of any subsequent experiences of victimization. When victimized later, for example, youth with program exposure more often expressed the belief that they were better able to protect themselves and mitigate the extent of any personal injury.

However small the differences were between youth who had participated and those who had not participated in a variety of the existing prevention programs, those who had the benefit of program exposure express the belief that they have, in fact, become better able to protect themselves and to keep abusive situations from becoming worse. Overall, these findings add to a growing consensus that involvement in school-focused programs with an array of prevention approaches is beneficial for children and teens. Based on this consensus, it has become a core part of Kayla's mission to use her personal story as an educational tool that can one day be integrated into a comprehensive CSA curriculum within schools and other youth-serving organizations.

Thus, while program-specific content and effectiveness can be difficult to study because the design of these school-focused programs varies considerably, in a comprehensive review in 2009 of the relative benefits of school-based abuse prevention programs, Keith Topping and Ian Barron at the University of Dundee, Scotland, concluded that they can be maximally effective if the following essential core components are in place:

- Their effectiveness can be evaluated.
- Modeling, discussion, and skills rehearsal are incorporated.
- They are at least four to five sessions long.
- They can be delivered by a range of personnel.
- Active parental input is encouraged.

Ideally these programs help youth not only learn the warning signs of grooming behavior but also practice the refusal skills they would need if they are ever in a situation where an adult began to touch them inappropriately. By having more than a one-time class or discussion, youth also report that they feel supported knowing that they could more easily talk to and call on these peers should they need to. And as far as implementation is concerned, school programs require relatively little supplemental funding as the curriculum is often adopted from materials available in the public domain and teachers can, with only brief training, learn to fold this topic into what is usually a broader wellness program throughout a school.

It is our hope that this book, featuring Kayla's candid revelations and the lessons that might be learned from them, will be an important addition to curricula around the country and worldwide geared toward greater awareness and prevention of this crime. Moreover, Kayla's personal narrative of childhood abuse along with her courageous transition from victim to survivor will serve, we believe, as a model for youth who remain afraid and ashamed and serve as an important example of how sexual abuse unfolds and can ultimately be combated.

COMMUNITY-BASED PREVENTION INITIATIVES AND ORGANIZATIONS

There have been a number of both publicly and privately funded community-based initiatives to stamp out CSA, and many employ comprehensive efforts that go beyond student-focused education alone. An example of this approach, the Comprehensive Sexual Abuse Prevention Education Act (CSAPEA), was introduced in Massachusetts in the 2015 legislative session and represents an adult-focused and policy-driven strategy designed to include, and go beyond, teaching educators about reducing the risk of CSA. It proposes building "adult and community responsibility" as a necessary first core element upon which policy can then effectively be developed. It recommends a hands-on, practical method for imparting critical information to students about the boundary-violating behaviors they, *and all the adults and children around them,* must watch for and report so that sexual exploitation never has a chance to take hold. Children, along with the adults who care for them, learn to identify the signs of child sexual abuse and steps that can be taken to interrupt possible abuse before it is fully set in motion by the perpetrator.

Initiatives like CSAPEA are rooted in the critical knowledge that children in the United States today are involved in many additional youth-serving extracurricular activities conducted by adults who, by virtue of their positions in these groups, have both the access and potentially the "cover" to engage in sexually inappropriate relationships with the children they serve. Included here are the over 35 million children who participate in youth sports programs as estimated by a 2015 *USA Today* survey done by Michigan State University. And although it is always difficult to obtain recent and consistent prevalence estimates as we have noted in earlier chapters, in 2004 a U.S. Department of Education report contained the then startling data that nearly 7%, or approximately 3.5 million of American school children, report having had unwanted sexual contact with someone in their school—usually a teacher or coach. This Department of Education finding shed more light on the magnitude of the problem and supported the contention of advocates and survivors that both school- and community-based prevention efforts were necessary not only to educate children who may be sexually abused in their own families, but also to reduce sexual misconduct and boundary violations by adults who are known to a child and abuse their power by engaging in sexual abuse.

Beyond the Massachusetts initiative, many other states, and now even the federal government, have enacted or are considering legislation geared toward increasing CSA awareness and prevention efforts through comprehensive school and community reform. Taken as a whole the key elements considered fundamental to these initiatives include mandates that cover:

- Schools and youth organizations
- Both public and private schools
- Awareness initiatives for elementary and secondary schools
- Adults and children (targeting adults as the first line of defense against CSA)
- Educating all school employees
- Preventing adult and child-on-child sexual abuse
- Responding to boundary-violating behaviors and reporting suspected cases
- Promoting organizational and safe-child policies and procedures
- Educating children about safe-child standards and giving them the related skills

Grasping the magnitude of this problem and the desperate need to educate adults in order to maximize the protection of our children across a spectrum of ages and sites, Kayla's hope is, here again, to use her public status and access to a diverse audience of adults to disseminate her message and personal experience as part of what is now a nationwide campaign to stop the scourge of CSA.

The Fearless Foundation

In addition to lending her voice to both established and fledging initiatives that have been described, Kayla has become aware through her personal experience of the importance of victims being able to re-experience their own strength and sense of mastery. Wanting to provide at-risk youth in particular with an opportunity to both learn and master new skills, and also benefit from her tutelage and story, Kayla established the Fearless Foundation in 2012.

Shortly before the 2012 Olympics I started speaking out and sharing my story. It was an amazing feeling to be so free from both my guilt and shame and the enormous pressure of knowing that now all eyes were on me. And it only got more intense. The day after I won the Olympics my phone would not stop ringing. Not with endorsement requests and sponsorship opportunities. No, that was not my problem. My mailbox was full with requests from schools, charities, organizations, Girl Scout clubs, churches, and survivor groups. My email was flooded with congratulations and pleas. Would I come speak to X's children's school? Would I come speak at the Boston Area Rape Crisis Center, where I had been a client? Would I speak in Cook County to a group of people who wanted to raise awareness? Would I lead a walk for healing and hope in Ohio? Would I talk to a survivor who was in pain? Could I give some advice to someone suffering from PTSD? It became overwhelming. And I felt an enormous sense of responsibility for these people. These victims. These survivors. They were me. And I wanted to help. So I started speaking anywhere and everywhere. I started taking calls and answering emails. I started traveling all over the country and sharing my story. But I was only one woman. And during these trips I noticed one common factor. There were SO many people who wanted to help. There were so many organizations and moms and teachers and volunteers who wanted to put an end to victims' suffering and bring forth healing and hope. But where do they go? How do they help? And so I realized my true purpose. The true reason for my journey and the gold medal at the end of that journey. The Fearless Foundation. I wanted to create something that will outlast medals and trophies and accolades. I wanted to create something that will outlast me. I wanted to create something that would change the world.

The mission of the Fearless Foundation is to shine a light on what child sexual abuse is and to help victims find healing and hope through mastery, ultimately helping them to become survivors. The first part of that is education. I want to educate our society about CSA. What it looks like, what it feels like, how you can stop it. And that is why this book came about. Eventually I want to create a curriculum for students in health class. I want them to have to read about it as they do about stranger danger and saying no to drugs. I want them to be educated as they are on bullying and safe sex. I want them to know what they can do and who they can talk to if someone close has tried to or has taken advantage of them. I want to create a way to change our society's taboo and ignorance on this topic. I want to have the conversation. A portion of the earnings from this book will go to funding the Fearless Foundation.

Once the curriculum is written I want to set up an online network for survivors. I want them to go to Google and type in abuse, and I want the website to pop up. I want them to be able to type in their zip code and get all the tools for healing. The rape crisis hotline. The place to go for pro bono therapy. The DA's number and the police officer they should talk to. An online support group for them to be free and safe to talk about their trauma and begin the steps toward finding the help they need.

I also want the foundation to help survivors find their mastery. For me it was judo. So I'm developing a program where survivors can come and take judo once a week from a SafeSport-approved coach and just be kids again. But eventually I want it to be more than judo. I want kids to find their passion. Maybe it's painting. Maybe it's archery. Maybe it's knitting. Whatever it is I want kids to be able to find a safe, healthy environment to be able to start reclaiming control of their lives.

This is my goal. And this is the goal of the Fearless Foundation. To take what was once my darkest moment and find the courage to *help others turn their darkest moment into a tipping point. I want to help them find the way out.*

To learn more about the Fearless Foundation, you can visit www.kaylaharrison.com.

One of the positive advances that we can note about the crime of child sexual abuse is that, unlike 20 years ago, there are now a multitude of organizations, campaigns, and programs that you can donate to or give your time to, all dedicated to its eradication. From the local level where you want to ensure that your school is taking steps to include information about CSA and mandate reporting in its curriculum, to the state level where you can join in efforts to expand community awareness and prevention, there are always ways to make a contribution. On the national and international level many public service campaigns are directed at eradicating CSA, and you can find out about the work they do by adding your name to some of the organizations listed in the Resources, such as RAINN (Rape, Abuse & Incest National Network), Prevent Child Abuse America, or GenerationFIVE, whose mission is to end child abuse within five generations through survivor and bystander leadership development. If you personally are a survivor who would like to know how to get involved, there are likely resources, organizations, and foundations that exist to help with your particular type of past abuse, including the Survivors Network of those Abused by Priests (SNAP) and INCITE!, which was organized to help women of color combat violence of all kinds both personally and within their community. Getting involved and speaking up is really what matters here, as it will take a pervasive culture change, starting in each home and community, for the scourge of CSA to end.

For all three of us, this book is so much more than a resource created to add to the existing educational materials on child sexual abuse; it is the culmination of a shared dream. As mental health professionals two of us have worked for decades helping survivors and their families, although sadly up to this time most of our work has promoted recovery and not prevention. By the time victimized children or teens cross our thresholds at McLean they have typically suffered for months if not years, and frequently we are the first people to hear their painful revelations. In these instances we have felt both frustrated and inadequate, wondering how we could possibly make more of a difference in reaching children and teens before they have been hurt and need to see us professionally.

Kayla's bravery and determination presented us with the opportunity to make a difference by combining our expertise with Kayla's narrative to help shape this cautionary tale, a tale we hope will reach parents, caregivers, educators, and youth alike. And if this story helps even one child and parent avoid the suffering of sexual victimization, the suffering endured by Kayla and countless others, then the three of us will have made the impact we hoped for.

Epilogue

When I was 16, I had what many would call a life-changing moment. I didn't realize it at the time or in fact for a long time after. But this moment comes to my mind so often now that I am where I am. And it comes to the forefront when I think about who I want to be or why life is so damn hard sometimes.

I had been training at the Pedros' for about 6 months. To say I was at rock bottom would be an understatement. Most days I didn't get out of bed, let alone chase my dreams. The best word I can use to describe me is numb. I was numb to the world. Numb to my friends, judo, my family, everything. I was just trying to survive.

We had to go to a competition called the U.S. Open. And at the time it was one of the bigger competitions I had fought in. So we as a team flew down. I made weight even though I was struggling with binge eating and maintaining a healthy lifestyle.

The next day in the competition I was a mess. I was scared and anxious and feeling very out of sorts. But one match at a time I found myself winning. I threw the first girl. And then I had a tough match but ended up beating the second girl on points. There were girls from all over the world in the division. Somehow, some way, I ended up in the finals of the U.S. Open.

They make a spectacle of it. There's lights and fog and an announcer. I remember being in the back warming up and feeling so . . . out of it. And then it was my turn. The announcer introduced my opponent and then me.

"From the United States of America, Kayyyyyyyylaaaaaaa Har-risonnnnnnnn."

I walked out on that mat, and I don't remember how or why, but I won. I won the U.S. Open. And my teammates are jumping up and down and the crowd is cheering, "USA, USA, USA!" And Big Jim is smiling and nodding his head. And all I remember feeling was completely empty. Hopeless. Like I would never be happy again. And that's when I decided I was done. I was going to quit. I couldn't do it anymore. But first I had to tell Big Jim.

So we flew home and I drove up to New Hampshire to his lake house. It was early morning, but he was already up and had worked out. He was sitting outside watching the sun and smoking his cigar. I joined him.

I gave him excuse after excuse. And reason after reason. I didn't want to be the strong girl. And I wasn't meant to be the golden girl. It was too hard, I was too tired. I couldn't do it. I quit.

And he listened to everything I had to say. And he let me cry and mope and cry some more. And when I was done, he said something that changed my life. He said:

"You know what, kid? What happened to you happened to you. And it's a terrible thing. But it doesn't define you. You're only a victim if you allow yourself to be. Now you've got a chance to go do something great with your life. But only YOU can decide."

And I sat there soaking it in. It doesn't define me. It **doesn't** define me.

And I said, "Okay, Big Jim, I'll see you at practice tomorrow."

It wasn't the flick of a switch; it wasn't a snap of a finger. But the next day I got out of bed and I brushed my hair. And then the next day after that I got out of bed and I brushed my hair, and my teeth. And then I went to practice. And school. And therapy. And then a year later I stood on top of my first world podium—Junior World Champion.

And looking back, one would say I have done many great things with my life. Junior world champion. World champion. Nine-time national champion. Our country's only and reigning two-time Olympic Champion. But those aren't the things that make me great. Those are not the great things that Big Jim was talking about. This is.

Writing this book has been the greatest thing in my life. Taking a stance and being Fearless has been the greatest thing in my life. Waking up every day and trying to be the difference I want to see in this world—that is the greatest thing I will ever do.

Life is always going to be hard. But we have a choice. We can decide. We can surround ourselves with lightness or darkness. We can choose to be around people who believe in us, before we even believe in ourselves. We CAN make a difference. And it all starts with a conversation. With one little first step.

I thank you for reading my story. I hope it has helped. I pray that it has shined a light on what is for many a deep, deep scar that we cannot see. I hope that this book allows those awful statistics to become just a little bit smaller. I hope we are all wiser and smarter about child sexual abuse. I hope that those victims who read this know: You are not defined by what happened to you. And you are not alone.

Resources

Organizations and Websites Offering Information, Support, and Resources on Child Sexual Abuse

United States

American Psychological Association
www.apa.org
The APA offers a page on sexual abuse under "Topics," which includes a definition of sexual abuse and more.

Assaulted Women's Helpline
www.awhl.org

Boys & Girls Clubs of America
www.bgca.org
The Boys and Girls Clubs promote safety for all children, including safety from sexual abuse.

Child Abuse Prevention Network (CAPN)
www.child-abuse.com
CAPN provides information on child abuse to parents, children, educators, and health care professionals, including statistics, prevention efforts, organizations and services, shelters, and news articles relating to child abuse prevention. This site also contains links to related information.

Child Welfare Information Gateway
www.childwelfare.gov

A service of the Children's Bureau, Administration for Children and Families, U.S. Department of Health and Human Services, the Child Welfare Information Gateway promotes the safety and well-being of children and families by providing information, resources, and tools on child welfare, child abuse and neglect, and more. It offers information on child welfare statutes and family support services along with print and electronic sources of information.

Darkness to Light
www.d2l.org

This is a nonprofit organization committed to empowering adults to prevent child sexual abuse. Offers resources for parents, organizations, survivors, and others, including a Stewards of Children Prevention Toolkit mobile app. Provides information such as risk factors for CSA, abuse reporting statistics, and *Child Sexual Abuse Disclosures: Guide for Practitioners*.

Fearless Foundation
www.kaylaharrison.com

Kayla Harrison's nonprofit organization dedicated to education about child sexual abuse and advocacy for victims.

GenerationFIVE
www.generationfive.org

A volunteer collaborative that seeks opportunities to promote a transformative justice approach to ending child sexual abuse in various locations across the country.

Joyful Heart Foundation
www.joyfulheartfoundation.org

The mission of the Joyful Heart Foundation is "to heal, educate, and empower survivors of sexual assault, domestic violence, and child abuse, and to shed light into the darkness that surrounds these issues."

Love Our Children USA
www.loveourchildrenusa.org/resources.php

A leading national nonprofit and prevention organization fighting all forms of violence and neglect against children in the United States.

MaleSurvivor
www.malesurvivor.org

This organization helps boys and men who have been sexually abused or victimized.

National Association of Adult Survivors of Child Abuse
www.naasca.org

A nonprofit organization in the United States and Canada dedicated to addressing issues related to childhood abuse and trauma, including sexual assault, violent or physical abuse, emotional traumas, and neglect through education and promotion of various paths to healing.

National Children's Advocacy Center
www.nationalcac.org

A nonprofit agency providing prevention, intervention, and treatment services to physically and sexually abused children and their families within a child-focused team approach. Resources and information for parents and professionals.

National Sexual Violence Resource Center
www.nsvrc.org

This group offers a variety of resources and sponsors April as Sexual Assault Awareness Month in the United States. The goal of SAAM is to raise public awareness about sexual violence and to educate communities on how to prevent it.

National Center on Domestic and Sexual Violence
www.ncdsv.org

The NW Network
www.nwnetwork.org

Support and resources for survivors of abuse who are lesbian, gay, bisexual, or transgender, through education, organizing, and advocacy.

Parents Anonymous (PA)
www.parentsanonymous.org

Promotes safety and resilience for families experiencing trauma, etc.

Pennsylvania Coalition Against Rape
www.pcar.org

PCAR works to end sexual violence and advocates for the rights and needs of sexual assault victims. It operates rape crisis centers throughout the state and operates the HERO Project, a public service campaign to spur adults to become a HERO for a child, providing them with the tools and confidence they may need to report suspected child abuse, including information on grooming behaviors.

Prevent Child Abuse America
http://preventchildabuse.org

With a network of 50 state chapters, this organization works to promote the healthy development of children and prevent child abuse before it can occur.

Rape, Abuse & Incest National Network (RAINN)
www.rainn.org

RISE: Roots for Individual & Social Empowerment
riseaboveabuse.org

Featuring a blog with personal stories shared by survivors of childhood sexual abuse as well as information on the legal aspects of dealing with the perpetrators of abuse.

Safe Horizon
www.safehorizon.org

The goal of this site is to help "victims of violence" transition from "crisis to confidence." Primarily serves the New York City area, but also helps those outside of the city find the support and resources they need.

Stop It Now!
www.stopitnow.org

This foundation based in Massachusetts prevents the sexual abuse of children by mobilizing adults, families, and communities to take actions that protect children before they are harmed. It identifies, refines, and shares effective ways for individuals, families, and communities to act to prevent child sexual abuse and to get help for everyone involved.

International Organizations

International Society for the Prevention of Child Abuse and Neglect
www.ispcan.org
A global organization that brings together a multidisciplinary group of professionals to work toward preventing and treating abused, neglected, and exploited children.

isurvive
isurvive.org
Created by survivors for survivors, this site offers resources and online support for people primarily in the United States, Australia, and Europe.

Australia

Rape & Domestic Violence Services Australia
www.rape-dvservices.org.au

Canada

Canadian Association of Sexual Assault Centres
www.casac.ca

New Zealand

Te Ohaakii a Hine—A National Network Ending Sexual Violence Together
http://toah-nnest.org.nz

South Africa

Shukumisa: Shaking Up Social Attitudes Towards Sexual Violence
http://shukumisa.org.za

We Will Speak Out South Africa
www.wewillspeakout.org/countries/south-africa

United Kingdom

End Violence Against Women
www.endviolenceagainstwomen.org.uk

National Society for the Prevention of Cruelty to Children
www.nspcc.org.uk
Offers a wide range of resources, services, research support, information, and more.

SurvivorsUK
www.survivorsuk.org

Rape Crisis England & Wales
https://rapecrisis.org.uk

Organizations Providing Information on Child Protection, Mandating Reporting Rules, and Other Statutes

National Center for Victims of Crime
https://victimsofcrime.org
Source of sexual assault statutes by state.

National Conference of State Legislatures
www.ncsl.org
Provides a detailed list of state statutes addressing child sexual abuse.
Also see Child Welfare Information Gateway, listed in U.S. organizations.

Organizations Offering Information on Treatment

American Association for Marriage and Family Therapy (AAMFT)
www.aamft.org

Association for Behavioral and Cognitive Therapies (ABCT)
www.findcbt.org

Behavioral Tech
https://behavioraltech.org
Offers a variety of resources for patients, families, and clinicians, including a directory of certified DBT therapists.

EMDR International Association
www.emdria.org

International Society for Traumatic Stress Studies
www.istss.org

McLean Hospital Residential Treatment Services: Adolescent and Young
    Adult
www.mcleanhospital.org/programs/3east

McLean's adolescent dialectical behavior therapy programs, collectively known as 3East, provide specialized care for teens and young adults who require treatment for depression, anxiety, PTSD, and emerging borderline personality disorder (BPD).

McLean's Adolescent Acute Residential Treatment (ART) program provides intensive, short-term, and highly-focused psychiatric care for teens and young adults through age 19 with emotional and behavioral difficulties, including youth with histories of trauma and PTSD.
www.mcleanhospital.org/programs/adolescent-art

McLean Hospital Residential Treatment Services: Adults

The McLean Hill Center for Women provides a safe, supportive, and secure environment to help women with trauma-related disorders build strength and find new resources to regain command of their lives.

Books

Fontes, L. A. (2015). *Invisible chains: Overcoming coercive control in your intimate relationship.* New York: Guilford Press.

Herman, J. L. (1997). *Trauma and recovery.* New York: Basic Books.

Pipher, M. (2005). *Reviving Ophelia.* New York: Penguin.

van der Kolk, B. A. (2015). *The body keeps the score: Brain, mind, and body in the healing of trauma.* New York: Penguin Books.

van der Kolk, B. A., McFarlane, A. C., & Weisaeth, L. (Eds.). (2012). *Traumatic stress: The effects of overwhelming experience on mind, body, and society.* New York: Guilford Press.

References

Chapter 1

American Psychiatric Association. (2013). *Diagnostic and statistical manual of mental disorders* (5th ed.). Arlington, VA: Author.

Conte, J. R., Wolf, S., & Smith, T. (1989). What sexual offenders tell us about prevention strategies. *Child Abuse and Neglect, 13*(2), 293–301.

Darkness to Light. (2015). Child sexual abuse statistics risk factors. Retrieved from *www.d2l.org/wp-content/uploads/2017/01/Statistics_4_Risk_Factors.pdf*.

The Hero Project; Pennsylvania Coalition against Rape. (2010). Retrieved January 29, 2017, from *www.pcar.org/parents-know*.

Kilpatrick, D. G., Saunders, B. W., & Smith, D. W. (2003). *Child and adolescent victimization in America: Prevalence and implications*. Washington, DC: National Institute of Justice.

National Center for Victims of Crime. (2017). Statistics on perpetrators of CSA. Retrieved July 27, 2017, from *https://victimsofcrime.org/media/reporting-on-child-sexual-abuse/statistics-on-perpetrators-of-csa*.

Snyder, H. N., & Sickmund, M. (2006). *Juvenile offenders and victims: 2006 national report*. Pittsburgh, PA: National Center for Juvenile Justice.

Whittle, H. C., Hamilton-Giachritsis, C. E., & Beech, A. R. (2014). "Under His Spell": Victims' perspectives of being groomed online. *Social Sciences, 3*(3), 404–426.

Chapter 2

American Psychiatric Association. (2013). *Diagnostic and statistical manual of mental disorders* (5th ed.). Arlington, VA: Author.

Carroll, M., Pfeiffer, S., & Rezendes, M. (2002, January 6). Church allowed abuse by priest for years. *Boston Globe Special Report.*

Henry, J. (1997). System intervention trauma to child sexual abuse victims following disclosure. *Journal of Interpersonal Violence, 12*(4), 499–512.

Herman, J. L. (1992). *Trauma and recovery.* New York: Basic Books.

Hershkowitz, I., Lanes, O., & Lamb, M. E. (2007). Exploring the disclosure of child sexual abuse with alleged victims and their parents. *Child Abuse and Neglect, 31,* 111–123.

London, K., Bruck, M., Ceci, S. J., & Shuman, D. W. (2005). Disclosure of child sexual abuse: What does the research tell us about the ways that children tell? *Psychology, Public Policy, and Law, 11*(1), 194–226.

Molnar, B. E., Buka, S. L., & Kessler, R. C. (2001). Child sexual abuse and subsequent psychopathology: Results from the National Comorbidity Survey. *American Journal of Public Health, 91*(5), 753–760.

Paine, M. (2002). Factors influencing children to self-disclose sexual abuse. *Clinical Psychology Review, 22,* 271–295.

Terr, L. C. (2003). Childhood traumas: An outline and overview. *Focus, 1*(3), 322–334.

Townsend, C., Rheingold, A., & Haviland, M. L. (2016). *Estimating a child sexual abuse prevalence rate for practitioners: An updated review of child sexual abuse prevalence studies.* Charleston, SC: Darkness to Light.

Chapter 3

Bacon, H., & Richardson, S. (2001). Attachment theory and child abuse: An overview of the literature for practitioners. *Child Abuse Review, 10,* 377–397.

Bolen, R. M. (2001). *Child sexual abuse: Its scope and our failure.* New York: Springer.

Hershkowitz, I., Lanes, O., & Lamb, M. E. (2007). Exploring the disclosure of child sexual abuse with alleged victims and their parents. *Child Abuse and Neglect, 31,* 111–123.

Malloy, L. C., Brubacher, S. P., & Lamb, M. E. (2013). "Because she's one who listens": Children discuss disclosure recipients in forensic interviews. *Child Maltreatment, 18*(4), 245–251.

McElvaney, R. (2008). *How children tell: Containing the secret of child sexual abuse.* Unpublished doctoral dissertation, Trinity College, Dublin, Ireland.

Schaeffer, P., Leventhal, J. M., & Asnes, A. G. (2011). Children's disclosures of sexual abuse: Learning from direct inquiry. *Child Abuse and Neglect, 35*(5), 343–352.

Sedlak, A., & McPherson, K. S. (2010). *Survey of youth in residential placement: Youth's needs and services.* Washington, DC: Westat.

Townsend, C. (2017). *Child sexual abuse disclosure: What practitioners need to know.* Charleston, SC: Darkness to Light. Retrieved from *www.D2L.org.*

Wilson, A. (2002, November 3). War and remembrance: Controversy is a constant for memory researcher Elizabeth Loftus, newly installed at UCI. *The Orange County Register.* Retrieved July 28, 2017, from *http://williamcalvin.com/2002/OrangeCtyRegister.htm.*

Chapter 4

Child Abuse Prevention and Treatment Act (CAPTA). (1974). Retrieved from *www.childwelfare.gov.*

Chapter 5

Allnock, D., & Miller, P. (2013). *No one noticed, no one heard: A study of disclosures of childhood abuse.* London: National Society for the Prevention of Cruelty to Children.

American Psychiatric Association. (2013). *Diagnostic and statistical manual of mental disorders* (5th ed.). Arlington, VA: Author.

Cook, A., Blaustein, M., Spinazzola, J., & van der Kolk, B. (2003). *Complex trauma in children and adolescents: White paper from the National Child Traumatic Stress Network, Complex Trauma Task Force.*

DeFrancis, V. (1969). *Protecting the child victim of sex crimes committed by adults.* Denver, CO: American Humane Association, Children's Division.

Lalor, K., & McElvaney, R. (2010). Child sexual abuse, links to later sexual exploitation/high-risk sexual behavior, and prevention/treatment programs. *Trauma, Violence, and Abuse, 11*(4), 159–177.

McNulty, C., & Wardle, J. (1994). Adult disclosure of sexual abuse: A primary cause of psychological distress? *Child Abuse and Neglect, 18*(7), 549–555.

Molnar, B. E., Buka, S. L., & Kessler, R. C. (2001). Child sexual abuse and subsequent psychopathology: Results from the National Comorbidity Survey. *American Journal of Public Health, 91*(5), 753–760.

Putnam, F. W. (2003). Ten-year research update review: Child sexual abuse. *Journal of the American Academy of Child and Adolescent Psychiatry, 42*(3), 269–278.

Ullman, S. E., & Filipas, H. H. (2005). Ethnicity and child sexual abuse experiences of female college students. *Journal of Child Sex Abuse, 14*(3), 67–89.

van der Kolk, B. A., Pynoos, R. S., Cicchetti, D., Cloitre, M., D'Andrea, W., Ford, J., et al. (2009). *Proposal to include a developmental trauma disorder diagnosis for children and adolescents in DSM-V.* Unpublished manuscript, the National Child Traumatic Stress Network Developmental Trauma Disorder Taskforce, University of California, Los Angeles, CA. Retrieved from *www.traumacenter.org/announcements/dtd_papers_oct_09.pdf*.

Chapter 6

Auerbach, R. P., Kim, J. C., Chango, J. M., Spiro, W. J., Cha, C., Esterman, M., et al. (2014). Adolescent nonsuicidal self-injury: Examining the role of child abuse, comorbidity, and disinhibition. *Psychiatry Research, 220*, 579–584.

Bohus, M., Dyer, A. S., Priebe, K., Krüger, A., Kleindienst, N., Schmahl, C., et al. (2013). Dialectical behaviour therapy for post-traumatic stress disorder after childhood sexual abuse in patients with and without borderline personality disorder: A randomized controlled trial. *Psychotherapy and Psychosomatic Medicine, 82*(4), 221–233.

Cloitre, M., Courtois, C. A., Charuvastra, A., Carapezza, R., Stolbach, B. C., & Green, B. L. (2011). Treatment of complex PTSD: Results of the ISTSS Expert Clinician Survey on Best Practices. *Journal of Traumatic Stress, 24*, 615–627.

Cloitre, M., Koenen, K. C., Cohen, L. R., & Han, H. (2002). Skills training in affective and interpersonal regulation followed by exposure: A phase-based treatment for PTSD related to childhood abuse. *Journal of Consulting and Clinical Psychology, 70*, 1067–1074.

Cohen, J. A., Mannarino, A. P., & Deblinger, E. (2006). *Treating trauma and traumatic grief in children and adolescents.* New York: Guilford Press.

Ehlers, A., Clark, D. M., Hackmann, A., McManus, F., & Fennell, M. (2005). Cognitive therapy for PTSD: Development and evaluation. *Behaviour Research and Therapy, 43*, 413–431.

Foa, E. B., Chrestman, K. R., & Gilboa-Schechtman, E. (2009). *Prolonged exposure therapy for adolescents with PTSD: Emotional processing of traumatic experiences: Therapist guide.* New York: Oxford University Press.

Harned, M. S., Korslund, K. E., & Linehan, M. M. (2014). A pilot randomized controlled trial of DBT with and without the DBT Prolonged Exposure protocol for suicidal and self-injuring women with borderline personality disorder and PTSD. *Behaviour Research and Therapy, 55*, 7–17.

Herman, J. L. (1992). *Trauma and recovery.* New York: Basic Books.

Krüger, A., Ehring, T., Priebe, K., Dyer, A. S., Steil, R., & Bohus, M. (2014). Sudden losses and sudden gains during a DBT-PTSD treatment for post-traumatic stress disorder following childhood sexual abuse. *European Journal of Psychotraumatology, 5*. [Epub ahead of print]

Linehan, M. (1993). *Cognitive-behavioral treatment of borderline personality disorder*. New York: Guilford Press.

Orsillo, S. M., & Batten, S. V. (2005). Acceptance and commitment therapy in the treatment of posttraumatic stress disorder. *Behavior Modification, 29*(1), 95–129.

Perry, B. D. (2009). Examining child maltreatment through a neurodevelopmental lens: Clinical application of the neurosequential model of therapeutics. *Journal of Loss and Trauma, 14*, 240–255.

Resick, P. A., Monson, C. M., Gutner, C., & Maslej, M. (2007). Psychosocial treatments for adults with PTSD. In M. J. Friedman, T. M. Keane, & P. A. Resick (Eds.), *Handbook of PTSD: Science and practice* (2nd ed., pp. 330–358). New York: Guilford Press.

Schneider, S. J., Grilli, S. F., & Schneider, J. R. (2013). Evidence-based treatments for traumatized children and adolescents. *Current Psychiatry Reports, 15*(1), 332–341.

Whitlock, J. (2010). Self-injurious behavior in adolescents. *PLOS Medicine, 7*(5), e1000240.

Zahl, D. L., & Hawton, K. (2004). Repetition of deliberate self-harm and subsequent suicide risk: Long-term follow-up study of 11,583 patients. *British Journal of Psychiatry, 185*(1), 70–75.

Chapter 7

Bass, E., & Davis, L. (2002). *The courage to heal: A guide for women survivors of child sexual abuse* (4th ed.). New York: HarperCollins.

Collishaw, S., Pickles, A., Messer, J., Rutter, M., Shearer, C., & Maughan, B. (2007). Resilience to adult psychopathology following childhood maltreatment: Evidence from a community sample. *Child Abuse and Neglect, 31*, 211–229.

Foa, E. B., Chrestman, K. R., & Gilboa-Schechtman, E. (2008). *Prolonged exposure therapy for adolescents with PTSD: Emotional processing of traumatic experiences: Therapist guide*. New York: Oxford University Press.

Lamoureux, B. E., Palmieri, P. A., Jackson, A. P., & Hobfoll, S. E. (2012). Child sexual abuse and adulthood-interpersonal outcomes: Examining pathways for intervention. *Psychological Trauma: Theory, Research, Practice, and Policy, 4*(6), 605–613.

Nooner, K. B., Linares, L. O., Batinjane, J., Kramer, R. A., Silva, R., & Cloitre, M. (2012). Factors related to posttraumatic stress disorder in adolescence. *Trauma, Violence, and Abuse, 13*(3), 153–166.

Rauch, S., & Foa, E. (2006). Emotional processing theory (EPT) and exposure therapy for PTSD. *Journal of Contemporary Psychotherapy, 36*(2), 61–65.

Chapter 8

American Medical Association. (1995). *Press release: The epidemic of sexual assault.* Chicago: Author.

Bernier, J. (2015). *State and federal legislative efforts to prevent child sexual abuse: A status report.* Chicago: Prevent Child Abuse America. Retrieved from *www.enoughabuse.org/images/FINAL-Published_PCA_MK_CSAstatus_report_9-2015.pdf Google Scholar.*

Child Maltreatment, 2014. (2016, January 25). Washington, DC: Administration for Children and Families, U.S. Department of Health and Human Services.

Collin-Vézina, D., Daigneault, I., & Hébert, M. (2013). Lessons learned from child sexual abuse research: Prevalence, outcomes, and preventive strategies. *Child and Adolescent Psychiatry and Mental Health, 7,* 22.

Comprehensive Sexual Abuse Prevention Education Act (CSAPEA), The Commonwealth of Massachusetts, Senate No. 316, Filed 1/15/2015. Retrieved from *https://malegislature.gov/Bills/189/House/H379.*

Douglas, E., & Finkelhor, D. (2005). *Childhood sexual abuse fact sheet.* Durham, NH: Crimes Against Children Research Center, University of New Hampshire.

Finkelhor, D. (2009). The prevention of childhood sexual abuse. *The Future of Children, 19*(2), 169–194.

Gibson, L. E., & Leitenberg, H. (2000). Child sexual abuse prevention programs: Do they decrease the occurrence of child sexual abuse? *Child Abuse and Neglect, 24*(9), 1115–1125.

Michigan State. (2015). Youth sports statistics. Retrieved from *www.statisticbrain.com/youth-sports-statistics.*

Minnesota Amateur Sports Commission, Athletic Footwear Association, USA Today Survey.

National Conference of State Legislatures. (2015). Child sexual abuse prevention: Erin's Law. Retrieved from *www.ncsl.org/research/human-services/erins-law-and-child-sexual-abuse-prevention-laws.aspx.*

Topping, K. J., & Barron, I. G. (2009). School-based child sexual abuse prevention programs: A review of effectiveness. *Review of Educational Research, 79*(1), 431–463.

Index

About the Authors

Kayla Harrison began training in judo at age 6 and is the first American to win an Olympic gold medal in the sport, which she did in both 2012 and 2016. Yet her competitive success masked an unimaginable personal struggle. At the age of 16, she revealed that she had been sexually abused by her coach for years. Today, Kayla uses her gold medal profile, voice, and example, as well as her Fearless Foundation, to encourage and empower other survivors of child sexual abuse. Now retired from competing in judo, Kayla is pursuing mixed martial arts with the Professional Fighters League. She lives and trains in Boston.

Cynthia S. Kaplan, PhD, is a faculty member at Harvard Medical School and Director of Trauma Training and Consultation in the Simches Division of Child and Adolescent Psychiatry at McLean Hospital. She has worked with numerous survivors of child sexual abuse and is coauthor of *Helping Your Troubled Teen*.

Blaise Aguirre, MD, is a faculty member at Harvard Medical School and Medical Director of the 3East Dialectical Behavior Therapy program at McLean Hospital. He treats many adolescents who have been sexually abused and is the author of *Borderline Personality Disorder in Adolescents: What to Do When Your Teen Has BPD*.